DEDICATION

RBC: To my family who gave me the time and encouragement to write a book and to the medical students who inspired me to translate my enthusiasm for microbiology into case presentations.

MGS: To my husband, Eric Bernstein, M.D. for his constant love, advice, support and inspiration, and to my children, Ali, David, and Kayla who remind me daily of how to find fun and excitement in learning something new.

KLM: To my parents, who taught me to reach for the stars . . . and to Pat, who loves and supports me every step of the way.

CONTENTS

INTRODUCTION

Over 20 years ago, Harvard Medical School began a major reform of their curriculum called the "new pathways to general medical education." Their original goal was to change how and what medical students were taught. The "new pathway" emphasized small group instruction, a self-directed approach to learning, and an integrated approach to the basic sciences and clinical experiences. Planning for the project began in 1982, and the new curriculum started in 1989. Since Harvard's initiative, over a dozen medical schools in the United States have made major changes in their curricula and their approaches to teaching medicine. While each is unique, the new curricula share many features, described below.

All have worked to integrate the basic sciences with clinical experiences. Under the traditional model, medical students spent the first two years in lecture halls and laboratories focusing on the basic sciences such as anatomy, biochemistry, microbiology, pathology, and pharmacology. The second two years were spent in clinical settings. With the new core curricula, clinical experiences start in the first month of medical school and continue for four years. In many of the programs, the basic science courses were shortened with the goal of revisiting the core concepts of the courses in the fourth year. In others, portions of the basic sciences are taught using clinical cases during the appropriate core clinical course. For example, concepts related to bacterial diarrhea are presented during a student's rotation in gastroenterology, and faculty who were once confined to lecturing in basic science courses now join a team of physicians so that clinical and basic science concepts can be integrated and taught together.

There is now a new emphasis on problem-solving skills. Major changes in healthcare demand that physicians approach problems in innovative and inventive ways. In small group sessions, the new curricula stress problem solving as practiced by clinical preceptors.

Under the new curricula, students spend more time in ambulatory and outpatient settings. The traditional model stressed clinical rotations in inpatient settings only. As more and more healthcare is delivered in an outpatient setting, this lets the classroom more appropriately reflect the current clinical experience. In some schools, students are matched with community physicians with whom they work for three years. This provides students a real-life perspective on chronic diseases as well as the role of primary-care physicians.

All of the programs allow students to explore new electives and self-directed study. Courses whose content includes medical ethics, clinical epidemiology, professionalism, physical diagnosis, medical economics, patient interviewing, population sciences, and health politics are appearing on medical school campuses for the first time. Lecture time at most schools has been shortened by 50%. This allows for an increase in the use of computer-aided courses and encourages students to acquire the skills and habits of self-instruction and to optimize their learning experience. In a number of schools, students have the option of a fifth or sixth year of study and have the opportunity to acquire an M.B.A., Ph.D., M.S., or law degree in addition to their M.D.

At many schools, there has been a shift from department-based courses to an approach based on individual organ systems. In an organ systems approach, when the heart and cardiovascular system are taught, all of the basic sciences involving the heart are taught at the same time. Such an approach requires the students to integrate the information in a very different way and avoids the redundancy that previously resulted from teaching each discipline as a separate course.

In summary, the new curricula have changed from being content-oriented to small group, case-based, interactive teaching. At the time this book was conceived, the authors were microbiology (RC, KLM) and infectious disease (MS) faculty participating in new curricula at their respective medical schools (University of Pennsylvania School of Medicine and Loyola University School of Medicine). Our goal was to create a case-based text that could be used by an integrated team teaching microbiology and/or infectious diseases. Our objective was not to attempt to cover every infectious disease or microorganism, but rather to use examples that would stress the key principles of microorganism pathogenesis, proper use of a clinical microbiology laboratory, and appropriate selection and use of antimicrobial agents. Because, sadly, many of the new curricula no longer include a laboratory component when teaching microbiology, we have tried to incorporate examples of material formerly stressed during microbiology labs. We have assumed that a faculty team including clinicians and basic scientists as well as students, residents, and fellows will be using this text and have tried to include case aspects such that every member of the team can participate. Each case has a patient history, differential diagnosis, clinical clues, laboratory data, pathogenesis, treatment and prevention, additional points, and references. The cases are presented as unknowns so that students will be challenged to create a differential diagnosis as they will in real life, making sure to include noninfectious causes that would present with similar clinical findings. Appropriate choice of lab tests needed to work through the differential diagnosis as well as instruction on specimen collection is included because these are areas that are rarely covered during core clinical rotations but that we believe to be incredibly important. Interpretation of laboratory results, pathogenesis, and treatment options are areas where we hope team members can participate in a discussion and dialog. Since different institutions have very different approaches, especially in their use of laboratory tests, we anticipate (and hope) that students and team members will debate many of the points presented as they work through a case. Because it is impossible to cover all organisms in this text, the "Additional Points" section (Section 1.7 in Case 1, Section 2.7 in Case 2, etc.) was created to impart microbiology and medicine key points that are important adjuncts to the case and related pathogens causing similar infections. The reference section proved a challenge for all of us because, like our students, we all actively use the Internet when challenged to review or look up critical information. For that reason, we have included Websites as well as review articles that we have all found to be helpful.

The cases are grouped by disease presentation from the simpler cases to the more complex. Each case can stand on its own since technical terms, images, and concepts are embedded into the individual case, thus allowing each course director the ability to pick and choose when a case is to be presented to the students. This book is not meant to be a comprehensive microbiology text. It is designed to fill a unique niche created by the new curriculum. It is our hope that this book will be a skeleton for interactive learning and that clinical faculty will supplement the cases with their own clinical experience and the basic science faculty may enrich the cases with their expert knowledge of the pathogen's structure and virulence factors. It is a dynamic text that will require updates for treatment and prevention as these evolve. We have tried to update each chapter as new information became available and to censor ourselves by restricting the contents to those essential for medical students who are overwhelmed by the amount of material they must assimilate.

SUGGESTED READING

KELLER, M. AND P. KELLER, *Making Harvard Modern: The Rise of America's University*, Oxford University Press, 2001.

THE ART OF DIFFERENTIAL DIAGNOSIS

A differential diagnosis is a list of possible causes of a patient's symptoms. More than just an itemization of diagnoses, however, it is a process or method that involves formulation of hypotheses, intuition, and validation or confirmation. The ability to generate a comprehensive yet targeted differential diagnosis for an individual patient is an important skill that involves the art as well as the science of medicine. It is a skill that improves with clinical experience and cannot be fully learned by reading textbooks alone. Although there are several computer models available that can generate a differential diagnosis in many areas of medicine, these models have not replaced the efforts of the skilled clinician.

It has been said in medicine that when patients present with illnesses, they often "do not read the textbook," meaning that there may be substantial variation in the presenting signs and symptoms in an individual patient compared to a textbook case. A corollary to this is that, in addition to common presentations of common diseases, there are both common presentations of uncommon diseases and uncommon presentations of common diseases. The expert clinician is alert to all of these possibilities.

The process of developing a differential diagnosis begins with the patient's initial complaint and is expanded with the history of the present illness and past medical history. Data from the patient's social history, including travel, exposures, sexual contacts, and living situation, may be particularly important in the field of infectious diseases. Often, the physical examination provides confirmation of the suspected diagnostic possibilities, and laboratory results can provide further evidence, or a final diagnosis. Part of the fun of medicine is the detective work employed in arriving at a differential diagnosis. The astute clinician must know which potential clues are important, which can be dismissed, and how best to prioritize all of the diagnostic possibilities. Empiric therapy may be directed at a variety of potential pathogens while awaiting a microbiologic diagnosis. The process of generating a differential diagnosis starts with a broad, inclusive list of possibilities, some of which are unlikely, to avoid the in advertent exclusion of the possible common presentation of an uncommon disease as well as the converse. Each added piece of clinical evidence allows you to narrow the differential diagnosis to a few possibilities that will direct the laboratory workup.

A common mistake is to not reconsider other possible diagnoses in the face of new data that do not support the initial provisional diagnosis. There must be flexibility in thinking even though there is a tendency to focus on confirmatory evidence and to dismiss contradictory evidence. It is, therefore, desirable for the differential diagnosis to evolve over time as more data about a patient become available and to even revisit possible diagnoses that may have been dismissed earlier in the process. Many students are first exposed to the art of differential diagnosis in clinical conferences where a student will present a difficult case to a seasoned clinician. The professor will often generate a differential diagnosis on the spot. Such a process is more akin to generating a "list" of possibilities rather than a demonstration of the necessary evolution of thought that occurs when one is faced with a real-life patient scenario.

There are several important principles in the art of differential diagnosis:

1. Be broad at first. Consider common and rare presentations of common and uncommon diseases. Although it is often said that "when you hear hoofbeats you should think of horses, not zebras," it is important to consider the zebras as well. To get you started, we have included a section for each case called "Clinical Clues." These "clues" are not meant to be exhaustive, but to highlight common associations that occur with common disease presentations. They are based on observations that you may make during the patient's physical exam and answers to epidemiologic questions you should ask when taking the patient's history. These clues may be helpful when you prepare your differential diagnosis.

2. Use each piece of data (presenting complaint, history of the present illness, past medical history, family and social history, laboratory results) to help you prioritize the differential diagnosis.

3. Don't be afraid to go back and ask questions later that you may not have considered initially. The differential diagnosis is a work in progress.

4. Ask all the important questions, such as those about travel, exposures to other sick persons, sexual history, occupation, and pets. It is often helpful to ask open-ended questions, such as "Is there anything else you would like to tell me," or "Is there anything I might have missed?"

5. Be cognizant of the fact that it is human nature to look for supporting evidence of a pet theory and to dismiss contradictory evidence. Keep rechecking your top few diagnoses with each new piece of clinical and laboratory data. Don't be "married" to your initial diagnosis.

6. Use your differential diagnosis to generate an efficiently prioritized laboratory workup. The speed at which this must be accomplished depends on the severity of the illness. You will not be faulted for ordering a multitude of tests on a patient who is critically ill and has a vague

constellation of signs and symptoms. For many patients, however, an initial negative evaluation may be followed by an observation period of "wait and see" to find out if something will "declare itself," rather than ordering numerous tests up front.

7. As Albert Einstein said, "Everything should be made as simple as possible, but not too simple." Enjoy the process!

ACKNOWLEDGMENTS

We want to acknowledge Marilyn A. Leet for her assistance with photography and Dr. Robert Jerris for sharing his virology images.

LIST OF COMMON ABBREVIATIONS

AIDS   –   acquired immunodeficiency syndrome
C   –   Celsius or centigrade
cm   –   centimeter
dL   –   deciliter
F   –   Fahrenheit
g   –   gram
h   –   hour
H_2O –   water
Hg   –   mercury
IM   –   intramuscular
L   –   liter
lb   –   pound
mg   –   milligram
min   –   minute
mL   –   milliliter
mm   –   millimeter
s   –   second
U   –   Unit
μg   –   microgram
μm   –   micrometer

Boy with Acute Pharyngitis

1.1. PATIENT HISTORY

The patient was a 6 year-old male who had been in good health with no significant medical problems. In late September he presented to his pediatrician's office with a complaint of sore throat, fever, headache, and swollen glands in his neck for the past 36 h. On physical examination (PE), he had a fever of 38°C (100.4°F), a red posterior pharynx, yellowish exudate on his tonsils, and multiple, enlarged, tender cervical lymph nodes (Fig. 1.1). There were no other pertinent symptoms.

1.2. DIFFERENTIAL DIAGNOSIS

This patient had acute pharyngitis, the painful inflammation of the pharynx and surrounding lymphoid tissues.

Infectious Causes

The major causes of pharyngitis in an immunocompetent host are bacterial and viral. Mycobacteria, fungi, and parasites do not cause acute pharyngitis in a normal host.

Medical Microbiology for the New Curriculum: A Case-Based Approach, by Roberta B. Carey, Mindy G. Schuster, and Karin L. McGowan.
Copyright © 2008 John Wiley & Sons, Inc.

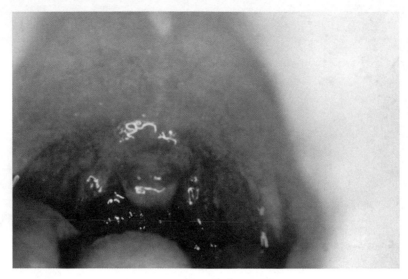

FIGURE 1.1 Acute pharyngitis.

Bacteria

Arcanobacterium haemolyticum—a much less common cause of pharyngitis seen predominantly in teenagers and young adults

Corynebacterium diphtheriae—rarely seen in the United States but should be considered with an appropriate travel history to Africa, Asia/South Pacific, South America, Haiti, Albania, and the former Soviet Republic countries

Mycoplasma pneumoniae—a cause of pharyngitis in teenagers and young adults

Neisseria gonorrhoeae—considered if suspecting child abuse

Streptococci, groups C and G—a cause of self-limited pharyngitis in young adults

Streptococcus pyogenes [group A strep (GAS)]—this is the most common bacterial cause of pharyngitis

Viruses

Adenovirus—causes pharyngitis, conjunctivitis, and acute respiratory disease

Epstein-Barr virus—causes infectious mononucleosis, which is seen predominantly in the 15–25 year-old age group and frequently starts with pharyngitis

Other respiratory viruses—rhinovirus, coronavirus, parainfluenza virus, influenza A and B viruses, coxsackievirus, cytomegalovirus

Fungi and Parasites

There are no agents in these categories that routinely cause acute pharyngitis.

[?] What is the age of the patient? Strep throat is usually seen in young school-age children.

[?] Does the patient have a runny nose and cold symptoms? Probable virus, not strep throat.

[?] Tonsillar exudates with fever and cervical lymphadenopathy and no cough? Classic signs and symptoms of *S. pyogenes* pharyngitis.

1.3. LABORATORY TESTS

A patient with GAS pharyngitis typically has a sore throat, fever, and pain on swallowing, as well as erythema with or without exudate on the tonsils and tender cervical lymph nodes. There are no clinical indicators that would make it possible to accurately predict the cause of this child's pharyngitis. Laboratory tests are required to make a diagnosis.

When deciding whether to perform a laboratory test, clinical and epidemiological features as well as the availability and usefulness of treatment must be considered. While viruses are the most common cause of acute pharyngitis in both adults and children, lab testing for viruses is not warranted because antiviral agents are not used to treat acute pharyngitis. Given the age of this patient, the absence of travel, and the lack of suspicion of child abuse, GAS is the most likely etiologic agent. Since GAS pharyngitis is the most commonly occurring form of pharyngitis for which antibiotic therapy is indicated, lab testing should be directed at ruling out GAS. Appropriate laboratory tests for this would include:

Rapid strep test. This is not a culture; the test detects a unique carbohydrate on the cell wall of GAS.

Throat culture. This test will grow the GAS organism from a throat specimen taken from the patient and will require overnight incubation at the minimum. Most labs offer a specific "rule out GAS" throat culture.

The specimen required for each of these tests is a throat swab. Use of a double-swab format allows one to obtain sufficient specimen to perform both tests if necessary. As with any microbiology test, the quality of the results is contigent on whether the laboratory receives a well-taken specimen. The double swab should be firmly rubbed over much of the surface of both tonsils and the posterior pharyngeal area and rolled to ensure that there is ample specimen is on each swab tip. If exudate is present, it should also be sampled on the same swabs. Care should be taken to avoid touching other areas of the oropharynx, mouth, and tongue.

Direct Gram stains from throat swabs are not at all useful because many bacteria normally reside in the throat, including nonpathogenic streptococci that have Gram stain appearance identical to that of GAS.

1.4. RESULTS

Rapid tests for detection of GAS directly from throat swabs are based on the detection of the group A–specific carbohydrate N-acetylglucosamine. While the sensitivity of these tests varies considerably, the specificity when compared to culture is excellent, ranging within 95–100% in most studies. For this reason, a positive antigen test is considered diagnostic of GAS and does not require throat culture confirmation. A negative antigen test result, however, must be confirmed with a throat culture. In comparison to most rapid tests, which take 5–10 min to perform, a throat culture requires 48 h to complete. The disadvantage of time delay when performing a throat culture has led to widespread use of the rapid antigen tests.

The rapid antigen test performed on one of the swabs obtained from this patient was negative (Fig. 1.2); the second swab was used to perform the throat culture. Culture of a throat swab on a single sheep blood agar plate is still the gold standard for confirming GAS pharyngitis. Assuming that an adequately collected specimen was submitted, a throat swab culture has a sensitivity of 90–95% for the detection of GAS. Once the swab is cultured, the plate should be incubated at 35–37°C for 18–24 h before reading. While many cultures will be positive after the initial overnight incubation, it is recommended that the plates be reincubated and examined again after another 24 h incubation. A considerable number of GAS do not appear until the second day and would be missed without the additional incubation time.

Streptococci demonstrate three types of hemolysis when grown on sheep blood agar: alpha (α), beta (β), and gamma (γ) (Fig. 1.3). α-Hemolysis is a result of incomplete destruction of red blood cells resulting in a green coloration of the media immediately surrounding the colony. β-Hemolysis

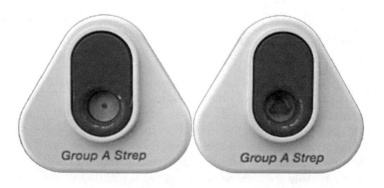

FIGURE 1.2 Rapid group A strep tests: negative (left), positive (right).

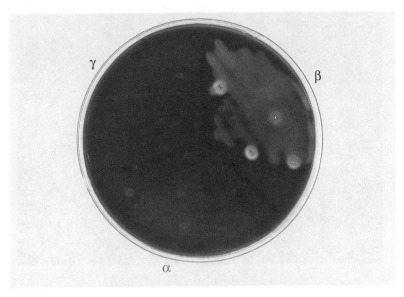

FIGURE 1.3 Blood agar plate with three types of hemolysis.

is complete lysis and destruction of the red blood cells resulting in a distinct clear zone around the colony. γ-Hemolysis is actually no hemolysis, and the result is the absence of a visible effect around the colony.

Group A streptococci are β-hemolytic and should show a distinct clear zone around each individual colony; however, not all β-hemolytic colonies are GAS, and further testing of β-hemolytic colonies is required. Even if a patient has GAS pharyngitis, many other bacteria representing normal colonizing flora will be present on the culture plate along with the GAS (Fig. 1.4).

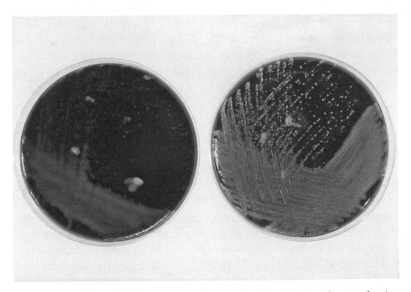

FIGURE 1.4 β-Hemolytic streptococci on selective (left) and nonselective media (right).

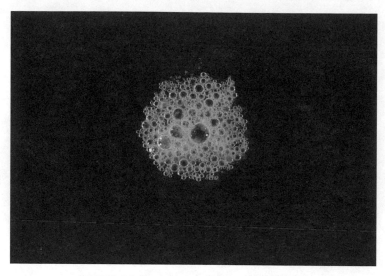

FIGURE 1.5 Positive catalase test (bubbles).

The plate is visually inspected for colonies that display β-hemolysis, and, if present, such colonies are further tested using the catalase test and a Gram stain for microscopic examination. The catalase test checks for the production of the enzyme catalase, using hydrogen peroxide as a substrate. A single β-hemolytic colony is mixed with a drop of 3% hydrogen peroxide on a glass slide, and immediate bubbling is seen if the test is positive (Fig. 1.5). Streptococci are gram-positive cocci in chains and are catalase-negative (no bubbles). In contrast, staphylococci (which can also display β-hemolysis) are gram-positive cocci in clumps or clusters and are catalase-positive. Gram-positive, catalase-negative cocci would then be further tested.

The bacitracin disk test provides a presumptive identification of GAS because >95% of GAS demonstrate a zone of growth inhibition around a disk containing the antibiotic bacitracin (Fig. 1.6). While this is a commonly used test in physician's offices, it requires another 18–24 h of incubation to perform. An alternative used by many clinical laboratories because it gives an immediate result is the PYR test, which detects the enzyme L-pyroglutamylaminopeptidase and can be performed within minutes using a single β-hemolytic colony. GAS are positive for PYR (Fig. 1.7).

The definitive method of identifying the β-hemolytic streptococci is by detecting the group-specific cell wall carbohydrate antigen directly from an isolated bacterial colony. These unique antigens classify the β-hemolytic streptococci into serogroups, designated by Dr. Rebecca Lancefield, as groups A, B, C, D, F, G, and so on. Kits containing group-specific antisera attached to latex beads are commercially available for this purpose and are used by many clinical microbiology laboratories. A single isolated colony is mixed with a drop of group-specific antibody, and if clumping of the coated latex particles occurs, it specifically identifies the serogroup.

The culture performed using the second swab taken from this patient was positive for β-hemolytic group A streptococcus (*S. pyogenes*). This is sufficient to confirm the diagnosis of GAS pharyngitis.

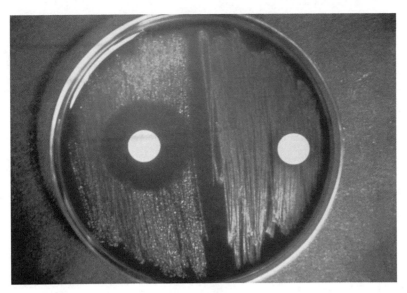

FIGURE 1.6 Bacitracin disk susceptible (left), resistant (right).

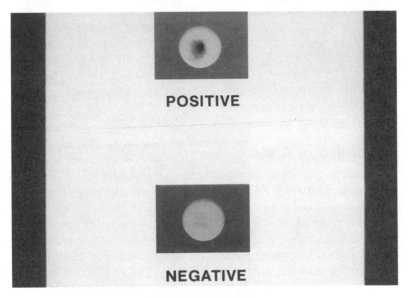

FIGURE 1.7 PYR tests.

1.5. PATHOGENESIS

Streptococcal pharyngitis is spread via aerosols from person to person, or less commonly by eating contaminated food. *S. pyogenes* is a successful pathogen since it possesses several virulence factors that allow it to invade tissue and escape host defenses. Some strains produce pyrogenic exotoxins, which cause serious systemic illness, such as toxic shock–like syndrome, which is associated with a high morbidity and mortality. The principal virulence factors produced by *S. pyogenes* are listed in Table 1.1.

TABLE 1.1.	*Streptococcus pyogenes* Virulence Factors	
Virulence Factor	Activity and Importance
M protein	Major virulence factor allowing bacteria to resist phagocytosis by host cells Appears as hair-like projections on cell surface >80 different serotypes Immunogenic (type-specific antibody is protective)
Streptolysin O	Hemolyzes red blood cells Activity destroyed by oxygen Immunogenic [antistreptolysin O (ASO) antibody formed during infection; can be used to diagnose recent infection]
Streptolysin S	Hemolyzes red blood cells Oxygen-stable Nonimmunogenic (no antibody formed)
Streptokinase DNases Hyaluronidase	Hydrolytic enzymes allowing bacteria to spread in host tissues Immunogenic (antibodies can be used to diagnose recent infection)
Hyaluronic acid capsule	Protects bacteria from killing by phagocytosis
Strep pyrogenic exotoxins (Spe A, B, C)	Cause release of host cytokines (interleukin, tumor necrosis factor), resulting in multisystem organ failure known as *toxic shock-like syndrome*

Infection with *S. pyogenes* may present in children as scarlet fever, which is fever and sore throat with a diffuse rash. The rash is caused by an erythrogenic exotoxin that has now been designated as one of the streptococcal pyrogenic exotoxins or Spe. The incidence of scarlet fever fell significantly in the 1950s largely because of the widespread use of penicillin.

The two major sequellae of untreated *S. pyogenes* infection, rheumatic fever (RF) and acute glomerulonephritis (GN), occur weeks after the streptococcal infection. The organism can no longer be cultured from the throat or skin when the patient presents with symptoms of RF or GN. RF occurs in <3% of people with strep pharyngitis. The patient presents with swelling and pain in more than one joint (migrating arthritis) and with a new heart murmur due to damage to the heart muscle and heart valves. The patient may also have a group of neurologic symptoms, including jerky or twitching movements (chorea). GN may occur 10 days or later after a skin infection with *S. pyogenes*. The patient has signs and symptoms of kidney dysfunction, such as swollen ankles and eyelids (edema), elevated blood pressure (hypertension), blood and protein in the urine, and decreased urine output. Deposition of antigen–antibody–complement complexes can be seen in a kidney biopsy using immunofluorescent stains.

The damage to the heart and kidney is not caused by systemic infection with the bacteria, but is theorized to be a result of direct damage by toxic streptococcal products (streptolysin O, streptokinase, and Spe) or an autoimmune response by the host. When the streptococcal bacteria are lysed by the host cells, antigens are released that evoke an immune response. Antibodies produced to the antigenic components of the bacteria cross-react with the patient's cardiac proteins, allowing the antibodies to attack the heart tissue and cause valvular damage. Later in life these damaged heart valves are a prime site where bacteria lodge and cause an infection of the heart known as endocarditis.

There is no antibiotic treatment for RF or GN; however, prophylactic penicillin is given to people with a history of RF to prevent recurrent streptococcal infections. Tests needed in the diagnosis of RF or GN may include antibody tests, such as antistreptolysin O or anti-DNase B to detect a recent infection after the viable organisms have disappeared. An acute (immediate) and a convalescent serum (drawn 14 days later) may be submitted for antibody titers to prove that the patient had a recent GAS infection. A fourfold rise in titer between the acute and convalescent sera indicates a recent infection, for example, an acute titer of 1 : 8 increases to 1 : 64 in the convalescent serum.

1.6. TREATMENT AND PREVENTION

Treatment of group A streptococcal pharyngitis is important in order to relieve the patient's symptoms and to prevent the transmission to others. Prompt treatment will also prevent complications such as peritonsillar abscess and acute rheumatic fever. Symptoms will often disappear within 3–4 days even without antibiotics, but early antibiotics can shorten the duration of symptoms. Pharyngitis caused by *S. pyogenes* can be effectively treated with a penicillin. In children, like this patient, amoxicillin is routinely prescribed. Patients must complete the course of antibiotic to eradicate the organisms from the pharynx. For patients who are allergic to penicillin, erythromycin would be an acceptable alternative. If left untreated, patients with GAS infection may develop the sequellae of heart valve damage (RF) or kidney damage (GN).

Susceptibility tests on GAS would not be performed since resistance to penicillin has not been documented in these organisms to date. Carriers maintain *S. pyogenes* in their throats despite appropriate antibiotic therapy; it is not because the organisms are resistant to penicillin. Carriers are not symptomatic but can spread the organism to others who may develop an infection.

1.7. ADDITIONAL POINTS

■ Who gets strep pharyngitis? A school-age child, 5–14 years old, would most likely become infected through contact with someone who carries the organism in their respiratory tract. While antibody does protect a person from repeat infection, the antibody is directed toward the M protein, and there are >80 serotypes of M protein, so that one can become infected with a different serotype again and again. Adults who have close contact with school-age children may acquire the infection more often. In adults, pharyngitis is most often the initial symptom of a viral illness that is accompanied by fever, runny nose, sneezing, and coughing.

■ While not widely in use, there are now molecular tests for the detection of GAS. Results from molecular testing can be available in less than 6 h, but since most labs perform the test once or twice a day, a more realistic turnaround time is 24 h. Negative molecular tests do not require culture confirmation, which saves time. Positive rapid tests (EIA) allow immediate results for the patients and physicians in busy emergency departments and clinics.

■ Infectious mononucleosis from Epstein–Barr virus (EBV) becomes more likely when clinical symptoms of rash, fatigue, hepatomegaly, and/or splenomegaly accompany the pharyngitis. If such were the case, then appropriate additional laboratory tests would include a complete blood count (CBC) and differential, and EBV-specific or non-EBV-specific serology tests. A relative lymphocytosis with an atypical lymphocytosis (>10%) is highly suggestive when combined with appropriate clinical findings. Nonspecific serologic confirmation would include a positive heterophil antibody titer or a positive Monospot slide test. A fourfold rise in antibody titer specific for EBV, or the presence of IgM antibody to EBV, serves as specific serologic evidence of recent infection.

■ Teenagers and young adults may develop pharyngitis with rash caused by a gram-positive rod, *Arcanobacterium haemolyticum*. This organism may resemble a β-hemolytic streptococcus on the culture media, but it is not a gram-positive coccus; it is a gram-positive rod. The organism will respond to most antibiotics used to treat strep pharyngitis.

■ Young adults, especially those of college age, may become infected with group C or G streptococci, which can cause an infection similar to that due to *S. pyogenes*. The rapid strep test will be negative since the group-specific carbohydrate is different in each Lancefield group. A throat culture will grow these organisms, but the physician may have to request further workup of these bacteria so that the group C or G strep is reported. Groups C and G streptococci are rarely associated with the sequella of GN and can raise ASO titers. The same antibiotic therapy for GAS may be given to relieve clinical symptoms and decrease transmission of infection.

■ Diphtheria is rarely seen in developed countries where healthcare practices provide for adequate immunization. A travel history to countries where diphtheria is endemic may require a throat culture for this organism. A gray membrane covering the posterior pharynx of a patient who lacks the common childhood immunizations should raise suspicions of diphtheria. The physician must notify the lab so that the appropriate media can be used to culture *Corynebacterium diphtheriae*.

SUGGESTED READING

BISNO, A. L., M. A. GERBER, J. M. GWALTNEY, E. L. KAPLAN, AND R. H. SCHWARTZ, Practice guidelines for the diagnosis and management of group A streptococcal pharyngitis, *Clin. Infect. Dis.* **35**: 113–125 (2002).

CUNNINGHAM, M. W., Pathogenesis of group A streptococcal infections. *Clin. Microbiol. Rev.* **13**: 470–511 (2000).

Red Book, *Report of the Committee on Infectious Diseases of the American Academy of Pediatrics*, 27th ed., 2006, pp. 610–620.

STEVENS, D. L., Streptococcal toxic shock syndrome: Spectrum of disease, pathogenesis, and new concepts in treatment, *Emerg. Infect. Dis.* **1**: 69–78 (1995).

Student with Dysuria

2.1. PATIENT HISTORY

A 20-year-old college student complained of burning when urinating and a strong desire to void frequently although she had little urine to void. She was not experiencing any pelvic pain or discharge. Her symptoms began shortly after she returned from a weekend visit to her boyfriend's school. She went to her university health service for diagnosis and treatment. On exam she was without fever and had moderate suprapubic tenderness, but no flank tenderness.

2.2. DIFFERENTIAL DIAGNOSIS

The patient presented with classic signs and symptoms of cystitis, an infection of the lower urinary tract, involving the urethra and bladder. Typical symptoms include pain on urination (dysuria), urinary frequency, urgency, and blood in the urine (hematuria). About 50% of women will have a urinary tract infection (UTI) during their lifetime. Dysuria may be observed with other infections such as vulvovaginitis or from numerous sexually transmitted diseases. Vulvovaginitis may be caused by a parasite (*Trichomonas vaginalis*) or a yeast (*Candida* species), or have a nonspecific etiology. Women with vaginitis complain of a malodorous vaginal discharge and dysuria and do not have urinary frequency or urgency. Women with urethritis have gradual onset of dysuria. Urethritis is typically caused by

Medical Microbiology for the New Curriculum: A Case-Based Approach, by Roberta B. Carey, Mindy G. Schuster, and Karin L. McGowan.
Copyright © 2008 John Wiley & Sons, Inc.

Neisseria gonorrhoeae or *Chlamydia trachomatis* and is a sexually transmitted disease. It is seen more commonly when there is history of a new sexual partner.

Since our college student did not present with vaginal discharge, she is more likely to have acute cystitis, which can be confirmed by a urine culture. Since she is an otherwise healthy woman and is not pregnant, her cystitis would be classified as uncomplicated cystitis. Risks for uncomplicated cystitis include being female, having sexual intercourse, history of previous UTI, and use of spermacide diaphragm contraception. A complicated UTI is one that involves the upper urinary tract or kidney. It is unlikely that her infection has progressed to pyelonephritis, an infection of the kidney and upper section of the ureter, since she had no fever or flank (lower back) pain. Risk factors for complicated UTI include male sex, pregnancy, anatomic or functional abnormalities of the urinary tract, diabetes, and immunosuppression. In the elderly patient, symptoms of UTI may be very subtle with loss of urinary continence and "smelly" urine without other classic symptoms.

Infectious Causes

In a normal host, the most likely cause of cystitis is bacteria from fecal flora that enter the urethra and bladder. Sexual intercourse increases the chance of bacteria entering the bladder. Uncomplicated cystitis is usually caused by one microorganism, *Escherichia coli,* but complicated cystitis may be polymicrobial. The majority of UTIs are caused by enteric bacteria that make up the normal gastrointestinal flora. Organisms include those listed below.

Bacteria
Enteric Gram-Negative Rods
> *Escherichia coli*—the most common cause of cystitis
>
> *Klebsiella* spp.—associated with hospital-acquired UTI
>
> *Proteus mirabilis*—associated with UTI and stone formation
>
> *Pseudomonas aeruginosa*—associated with hospital-acquired UTI
>
> Other gram-negative rods—depending on the patient's underlying condition

Gram-Positive Cocci
> *Enterococcus* spp.—more often associated with institutionalized patients (hospital, nursing home) rather than being community-acquired
>
> *Staphylococcus saprophyticus*—common agent of cystitis in young, sexually active females
>
> *Streptococcus agalactiae* (group B strep)—may cause infection in pregnant women

Viruses
> Adenovirus—causes hemorrhagic cystitis in children

Fungi

Candida spp.—causes UTI in diabetics, immunocompromised patients, and those with an indwelling catheter

Parasites

Schistosoma haematobium eggs—seen in urine sediment, found in those with travel history

Mycobacteria

Mycobacterium tuberculosis—may be shed in urine when infection is elsewhere in the body but is not a primary cause of UTI

CLINICAL CLUES

[?] Does the patient urinate frequently with little urine output? Typical symptom for acute cystitis.

[?] Presence of fever and flank pain? Suggest kidney involvement (pylonephritis).

[?] Is the patient a sexually active female? Most UTIs occur in young, sexually active females. A history of a new sexual partner suggests urethritis with *Neisseria gonorrhoeae* (GC) or *Chlamydia trachomatis*.

[?] Male patient with symptoms of cystitis? Cystitis is uncommon in men. If it's a recurrent UTI, suspect prostatitis.

2.3. LABORATORY TESTS

Urine Dipstick

A urine specimen was collected from this patient by a noninvasive technique, a midstream clean catch. Screening tests can predict which urine specimens contain a high colony count of bacteria. The most frequently used screening test with urine is called a "dipstick test". A dipstick consists of plastic strips that contain multiple pads with chemical indicators. Normal urine is sterile, without protein, white cells, blood, or nitrites. A positive test for nitrites indicates the presence of bacteria that produce nitrate reductase, changing nitrate to nitrite. A positive test for leukocyte esterase indicates the presence of polymorphonuclear neutrophils (PMNs) in the urine that produce the enzyme. Inflammatory cells are the host's response to infection. The strip is dipped into the urine, and the indicator pads turn colors that are read immediately and compared to a scale of +1 to +4 (Fig. 2.1).

A dipstick test performed at the university health center on the urine from our college student showed positive reactions for both nitrate and leukocyte esterase, so her urine was sent to the lab for culture. A urine culture should be performed in patients with suspected cystitis regardless of dipstick results.

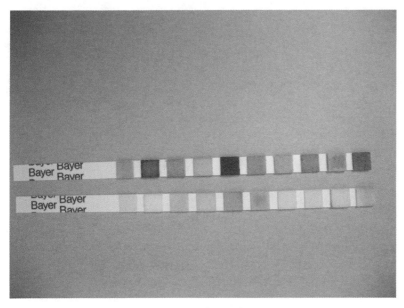

FIGURE 2.1 Urine dipstick reactions.

Urinalysis (Microscopic Exam)

Urinalysis to look for pyuria (WBCs in urine) and hematuria (RBCs in urine) should be performed on all patients suspected of having a complicated UTI. In addition, it may be useful to demonstrate pyuria in patients with clinical evidence of UTI but whose urine gives a negative dipstick result. All patients with acute cystitis should manifest ≥ 10 WBC/mm^3 in an uncentrifuged urine specimen. The finding of WBC casts in the urine indicates an upper tract infection (Fig. 2.2).

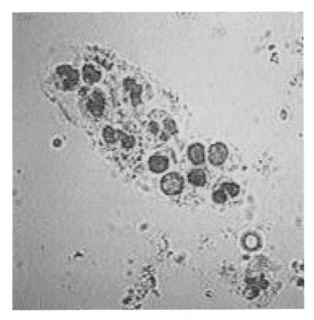

FIGURE 2.2 Urine WBC cast.

Urine Culture

To obtain a clean-catch urine for culture, patients should be instructed to clean the urogenital area well with soap and water three times, then begin to void, and in the middle of voiding, a portion of the urine should be collected into a sterile container. If a patient is unable to provide a good midstream urine, a catheter can be inserted into the bladder to obtain a specimen, but this technique is more risky for the patient since organisms may be introduced into the bladder during the procedure. In infants, a suprapubic aspirate can also be obtained by tapping the bladder with a needle and syringe.

Urine is terrific culture media, so once collected, it must be delivered immediately to the lab for testing, kept refrigerated, or placed in transport tubes with preservative. Urine that sits at room temperature for as little as an hour may yield false-positive results in screening tests and exhibit an increased number of bacteria in the culture, due to the multiplication of microorganisms after the specimen was collected.

Urine submitted for culture is inoculated onto several agar plates appropriate for recovery of both gram-positive cocci and gram-negative rods. The urine is inoculated with a calibrated loop that delivers a volume of 0.001 or 0.01 mL. The number of colonies is then multiplied by the dilution factor to provide a total colony count per milliliter of urine. Urine is one of the few specimens where quantitative results are given. Normal urine should be sterile. If $>10^5$ colony-forming units (CFU) of bacteria/mL are present, the patient is considered to have a UTI and the organism is identified and susceptibility testing is done. If more than three organisms are present in the same quantity, the urine is considered to be contaminated by normal urogenital flora and no workup is performed since no true pathogen has been found.

2.4. RESULTS

The urine culture from our college student showed greater than 100 colonies on the blood agar plate and the MacConkey agar, which selectively grows gram-negative rods. Multiplying the actual colony count by 1000, the total colony count is $>10^5$/mL and is clinically significant. The bacteria that grew on the MacConkey agar are pink, indicating that they are lactose fermenters (Fig. 2.3). Members of the family *Enterobacteriaceae* that ferment lactose are *E. coli*, *Klebsiella*, and *Enterobacter*. A spot indole test was positive (Fig. 2.4), indicating that the most likely pathogen in her urine was *E. coli*, and not *Klebsiella* or *Enterobacter*. A complete biochemical battery may be performed to confirm the identification.

Susceptibility test results showed our college student's *E. coli* to be susceptible to ampicillin, cefazolin, ciprofloxacin, nitrofurantoin, and trimethoprim–sulfamethoxazole (SXT), all of which can be given as oral preparations to an outpatient. The test was performed by disk diffusion in which a standardized amount of the bacteria are grown on a Mueller–Hinton agar with various antimicrobial disks overnight (Fig. 2.5). The diameter of the zone of inhibition around each disk is measured and interpreted as susceptible, intermediate, or resistant.

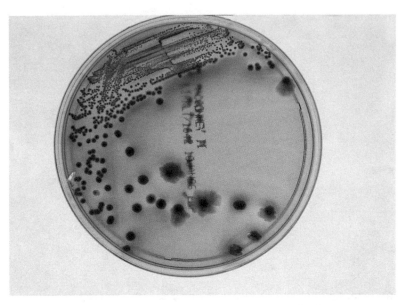

FIGURE 2.3 Lactose fermenting colonies on MacConkey agar.

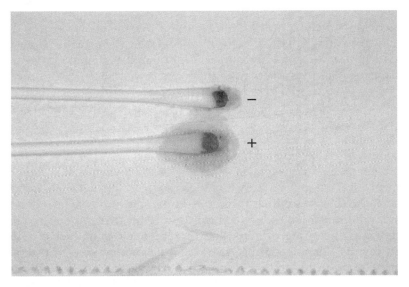

FIGURE 2.4 Positive blue-green indole reaction (bottom) and negative reaction (top).

2.5. PATHOGENESIS

Urinary tract infections are more common in women than men in all age groups except the neonatal period. With both men and women, the incidence of UTI rises with age. There are symptomatic and asymptomatic UTIs. Because some patients will have no symptoms, urine screening and urine culture are critical for detection. In the most serious cases, UTI can progress to sepsis.

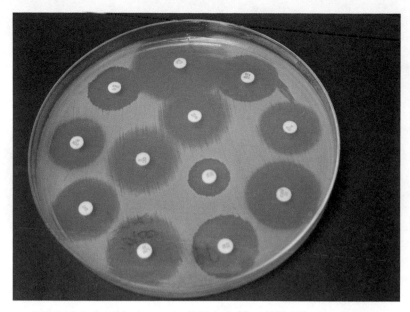

FIGURE 2.5 Antibiotic susceptibility test by disk diffusion method.

A wide variety of factors predispose a person to acquire a UTI. In infants and young children, congenital anatomic abnormalities are associated with UTI. Sexual intercourse, diaphragm use, diabetes, pregnancy, reflux, neurologic dysfunction, renal stones (urolithiasis), and tumors all predispose to UTI. In a hospital, nursing home, or homecare setting, indwelling catheters and instrumentation of the urinary tract are major factors contributing to UTI.

Infection of the urinary tract occurs via two major routes: either as an ascending infection or by a hematogenous infection. The most common way is the ascending infection, where enteric bacteria first colonize the perineum and anterior urethra, and then move up the urethra to infect the bladder and then sometimes further ascend to the kidneys. Infection with enteric gram-negative rods is almost always by this route. The second route involves seeding of the kidney during bacteremia (bacteria in the bloodstream). Renal infections due to *Staphylococcus aureus*, *Streptococcus pyogenes* (group A streptococci), and other bacteria that rarely cause cystitis are a result of this mechanism. Hematogenous infections are also the major cause of renal abscesses.

A number of virulence factors are responsible for *E. coli* and other enteric gram-negative rods as the predominant uropathogens in humans. Fimbriae are hair-like appendages on the surface of many gram-negative bacilli and some gram-positive species. There are hundreds of fimbriae on the cell wall of a single bacterium, and they are used for attachment to a variety of surfaces, including human cells. The attachment of bacteria to specific receptor sites on host cells within the urinary tract is the first step toward infection. Enteric bacteria attach to and colonize the perineum and anterior urethra prior to ascension into the bladder. The anatomically shorter and wider urethra in females is thought to account for the higher incidence of UTI in women. Further dilation of the urethra due to hormonal influence is responsible for the high incidence of UTI during pregnancy. Specific groups of fimbriae (type 1, P, S, F1C) are considered virulence factors for UTI. Production of type 1 fimbriae is considered the single most commonly expressed virulence factor in *E. coli* cystitis; P fimbriae are the second most common and associated with pyelonephritis.

Strains of *E. coli* produce capsular or envelope antigens called *K antigens*. Specific K antigens (K-2a, K-2c) are associated with *E. coli* strains that cause cystitis and also pyelonephritis. Research studies indicate that the quantity of K antigen produced, and not merely its presence, determines the virulence of a specific *E. coli* strain. *E. coli* that cause pyelonephritis produce 3–5 times the amount of K-2a and K-2c antigens than do *E. coli* strains that cause cystitis alone. Organisms that produce K antigens are less susceptible to killing following ingestion by phagocytic cells. In addition, K antigens allow bacterial strains to resist the bacteriocidal activity of immunoglobulins and complement in human serum.

Escherichia coli and other *Enterobacteriaceae* possess flagella for purposes of motility. It is believed that flagella are a contributing virulence factor helping bacteria swim upstream to the kidneys, causing pyelonephritis. Iron acquisition is an important virulence factor. Uropathogenic *E. coli* strains contain aerobactin, an iron-chelating protein that enhances survival of the bacteria in an iron-poor environment of body fluids.

Strains of *E. coli* that cause UTI carry large blocks of genes within their DNA called pathogenicity islands (PIs) that are not found within the genomes of nonuropathogenic strains of *E. coli*. Genes that code for virulence factors such as fimbriae, hemolysins, capsule synthesis, iron uptake, and toxins are all located on PIs. Uropathogenic strains of *E. coli* possess genomes that are 20% larger than the genomes of nonpathogenic fecal strains of *E. coli*. The PIs are thought to account for this genomic size difference. This suggests that there are many more pathogenesis and virulence genes yet to be discovered.

2.6. TREATMENT AND PREVENTION

Factors to consider when treating UTI include:

- Patient's age and sex
- Symptomatic versus asymptomatic infection
- Upper (pyelonephritis) versus lower (cystitis) urinary tract involvement
- Community- versus hospital-acquired infection
- Single event versus recurrent events
- Patient's underlying illness

For uncomplicated cystitis a 3-day course of treatment is recommended. Symptoms usually resolve over 1–3 days. Many antibiotics with a broad range of activity against gram-negative rods and/or gram-positive cocci are suitable for the treatment of UTI, whether they are bacteriostatic or bacteriocidal drugs because they are concentrated 10–30-fold in the urine. Choices for initial empiric treatment of uncomplicated UTI in women include trimethoprim–sulfamethoxazole, a fluoroquinolone, or nitrofuran-toin. The choice of an empiric antibiotic should always be based on the local prevalence of resistance in one's geographic area, and this should be periodically reevaluated. Ampicillin, amoxicillin, and sulfonamides are no longer considered good empiric choices because of the higher resistance rates seen in *Enterobacteriaceae* and *Enterococcus* spp. isolated from adults.

Follow-up urine cultures are not necessary for patients with uncom-plicated cystitis who respond clinically to treatment. Pregnant women should receive a follow-up culture 1–2 weeks after treatment. Compli-cated UTIs are more often caused by bacteria that may be resistant to the antibiotics used to treat uncomplicated UTI, particularly in hospitalized patients. Until the results of urine cultures are available in these patients, a fluoroquinolone is an excellent antibiotic choice in adult patients. In these patients, treatment should be continued for 7–14 days. If symptoms resolve, a follow-up urine culture is not generally recommended.

2.7. ADDITIONAL POINTS

■ A Gram stain of freshly voided urine, not concentrated by centrifu-gation, correlates well with a quantitative urine culture and can yield faster results. The finding of one bacterium or more per oil immersion field correlates with $\geq 10^5$ CFU/mL.

■ Lower colony counts ($<10^5$ CFU/mL) can be significant in females who are symptomatic; this is called *acute urethral syndrome*. It is important for the physician to communicate with the laboratory regarding the patient's status so that these urine cultures can be appropriately worked up.

■ If two organisms are present at $>10^5$ CFU/mL, they may both play a role in causing infection. Polymicrobial bacteriuria is common in the institutionalized elderly and those with complicated urinary tract infec-tions.

■ *Sterile pyuria* is a term that refers to the presence of WBCs in urine with no organisms recovered on bacterial culture. When this occurs in patients, one should consider anaerobes or fastidious organisms, such as *Neisseria gonorrhoeae*, as the possible causative agent. Not all bacterial causes of UTI are recoverable on the media routinely used to evaluate urine specimens. In such cases, one should consult with the laboratory.

■ A number of bacteria, most notably *Proteus* spp., produce the enzyme urease, which hydrolyzes urea to ammonia and carbamate and creates a high pH (>7). This alkalization of the urine decreases the solubility of calcium, resulting in precipitation of calcium and the formation of calcium urinary stones. *Proteus* species are commonly recognized in bacterial cultures because the colonies spread out ("swarm") over the agar media beyond the actual edge of the colony (Fig. 2.6).

■ A *Foley catheter* is an indwelling catheter that is held in the bladder by a balloon that is inflated with either air or liquid. Within 48 h following insertion, Foley catheters become colonized with bacteria, and posi-tive culture results seldom reflect bladder infection. Indwelling bladder

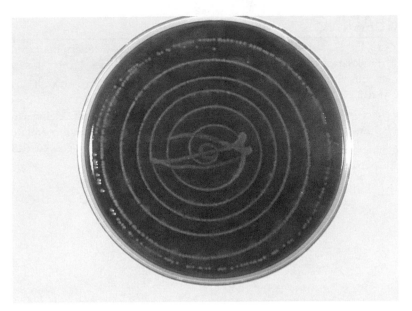

FIGURE 2.6 Colonies of swarming *Proteus*.

catheters do increase the risk of nosocomial (hospital-acquired) UTI. Diagnosis of UTI in this setting requires assessment of the patient's clinical status and the degree of pyuria and bacteruria.

■ *Trichomonas vaginalis*, a sexually transmitted parasite, can be detected in the microscopic examination of urine sediment as part of a routine urinalysis; however, *Trichomonas* is not a primary urine pathogen.

■ UTI in men is rare and must be distinguished from other syndromes. Men between the ages of 15 and 30 years who present with dysuria usually have urethritis, with or without urethral discharge. Men ≥40 years of age who present with dyuria, frequency, and urgency usually have inflammation of the prostate (prostatitis). Urinalysis and urine culture should be performed in both groups as part of the evaluation.

■ Additional renal function tests should be performed in all patients suspected of having pyelonephritis. These would include serum creatinine, blood urea nitrogen (BUN), and a microscopic examination of urine sediment. There is no microbiology test that can distinguish pyelonephritis from cystitis. It is diagnosed on the basis of clinical symptoms, which usually include fever and tenderness at the flanks or costovertebral angles along with pyuria and a positive urine culture. Finding WBC casts on microscopic urinalysis is also a helpful clue.

■ Other tests that may be useful in checking for structural abnormalities (infants and children), urinary reflux, or urinary obstruction are the intravenous pyelogram (IVP), in which a high-contrast medium are administered by intravenous injection followed by an x-ray of the renal pelvis and ureter, and the renal ultrasound. These tests should be considered in patients who have known preexisting urinary tract abnormalities, or in patients who do not respond to adequate antimicrobial therapy.

SUGGESTED READING

HOOTON, T. M., D. SCHOLES, J. P. HUGHES, ET AL., A prospective study of risk factors for symptomatic urinary tract infection in young women, *New Engl. J. Med.* **335**: 468–474 (1996).

KUNIN, C. M., *Urinary Tract Infections*, 5th ed., Williams & Wilkins, Baltimore, 1997.

NICKEL, J. C., Management of urinary tract infections: Historical perspective and current strategies: Part 2—Modern management, *J. Urol.* **173**: 27–32 (2005).

NICOLLE, L. E., S. BRADLEY, R. COLGAN, J. C. RICE, A. SCHAEFFER, AND T. M. HOOTON, Infectious Diseases Society of America guidelines for the diagnosis and treatment of asymptomatic bacteriuria in adults, *Clin. Infect. Dis.* **40**: 643–654 (2005).

Boy with Vomiting and Diarrhea after a School Picnic

3.1. PATIENT HISTORY

A 14-year-old male presented to his pediatrician for evaluation of vomiting, abdominal discomfort, and nonbloody diarrhea. Three days prior, he attended his school picnic, where he ate everything offered: barbecued chicken, potato salad, baked beans, tossed salad, and ice cream. Within 36 h of the picnic he noted mild abdominal discomfort, intermittent crampy abdominal pain, and three to five loose, watery bowel movements per day. He reported no blood in the stool, rash, pain on urination (dysuria), or blood in the urine (hematuria) and had no travel history, had no pets, and denied taking antibiotics. The school reports that at least 50 other students who attended the picnic are also reporting similar symptoms. On physical examination, he had a temperature of 39°C (102°F) and had normal vital signs. The abdominal exam was notable for mild lower abdominal tenderness. Other than his complaint of diarrhea, he is a healthy adolescent with no significant medical history. The fecal exam demonstrated a watery stool that was negative for occult blood.

3.2. DIFFERENTIAL DIAGNOSIS

This young man has acute diarrhea. Diarrhea is defined as abnormal frequency, fluidity, and/or volume of bowel movements. By definition, acute diarrhea continues for ≤14 days; persistent diarrhea, for >14 days; and

Medical Microbiology for the New Curriculum: A Case-Based Approach, by Roberta B. Carey, Mindy G. Schuster, and Karin L. McGowan.
Copyright © 2008 John Wiley & Sons, Inc.

chronic diarrhea, for ≥30 days. The differential for acute diarrhea would include bacterial or viral inflammation of the stomach and intestines (gastroenteritis), food poisoning that will usually resolve in 24–36 h, antibiotic-associated diarrhea, or noninfectious causes. Because of the association with a school picnic and evidence of a cluster of cases, an infectious cause such as bacterial or viral gastroenteritis is most likely.

Infectious Causes

Specific agents associated with acute diarrhea in a normal host include those listed below.

Bacteria

Aeromonas hydrophila

Campylobacter spp. (specifically *C. jejuni*)

Clostridium difficile

Escherichia coli [enterotoxigenic (ETEC), enterohemorrhagic (EHEC), enteropathogenic (EPEC), enteroaggregative (EAEC), and enteroinvasive (EIEC) strains]

Plesiomonas shigelloides

Salmonella spp. (*S. typhi* and nontyphoid strains)

Shigella spp.

Vibrio cholera

Vibrio parahaemolyticus

Yersinia enterocolitica

Viruses

Adenovirus (enteric)

Astrovirus

Norwalk virus (calcivirus)

Rotavirus

Parasites

Cryptosporidium parvum

Cyclospora cayetenensis

Entamoeba histolytica

Giardia lamblia

Fungi and Mycobacteria

There are no agents in these categories that routinely cause acute diarrhea in a normal host.

Noninfectious Causes

Crohn's disease

Diverticulitis

Inflammatory bowel disease

Milk protein intolerance (more frequently seen in infants)

Poisons

Ulcerative colitis

Risk Factors

Knowing specific pieces of patient information can be critical in identifying the cause of the patient's diarrhea. The history of a patient's illness can give important clues to the etiology. The risk of acquiring a gastrointestinal infection can vary with age, living conditions, geographic location, travel history, food habits, antibiotic use, attendance at daycare, and other factors. It is also helpful to know whether it is a single sporadic case of diarrhea or affects an entire household, or worse, everyone at a school or a company picnic, signaling a possible outbreak. It is very important that if you know such critical information about a person, you pass that information on to the laboratory attempting to isolate the possible pathogen(s). Certain epidemiologic associations are well known for organisms causing gastroenteritis (see Table 3.1).

CLINICAL CLUES

? Fever and/or bloody diarrhea? Suggests an invasive bacterial gastroenteritis such as *Salmonella*, *Shigella*, or *Campylobacter*.

? Nausea and vomiting a prominent feature? Viral gastroenteritis, ETEC, or EHEC are more likely.

? Current or recent antibiotic course? Suspect *Clostridium difficile*.

? Abrupt onset of nausea, vomiting, and diarrhea with no fever and quick resolution? A preformed toxin, such as *Staphylococcus aureus* enterotoxin.

3.3. LABORATORY TESTS

There are various interpretations of what is considered medically indicated for evaluating persons with acute diarrhea. Because most diarrheal illness is self-limited, the usefulness of stool cultures is questioned by some; however, early diagnosis can lead to interventions that both alleviate symptoms and prevent secondary transmission, which can have tremendous public health impact. In addition, detection of specific agents aids in the timely detection and control of outbreaks. Some causes of acute diarrhea can result in serious long-term sequelae such as Guillain–Barré syndrome (with *Campylobacter*) or hemolytic uremic syndrome (HUS) due to EHEC, further justifying the need for performing stool culture. A stool specimen for culture should be obtained as early in the course of the disease as possible from all patients with bloody diarrhea, patients with fever, in persons with diarrhea who are immunosuppressed, from patients in whom the diagnosis of HUS is suspected, and from persons involved in possible outbreaks.

| TABLE 3.1. | Organisms Associated with Gastroenteritis |

Organism	Association
Bacteria	
Aeromonas hydrophila	Consumption of untreated water, seafood
Campylobacter jejuni	Contaminated poultry or water, unpasteurized milk, contact with puppies or kittens
Clostridium difficile	Antibiotic use, the most common cause of acute diarrhea in hospitalized patients
Escherichia coli	
EIEC	Contaminated food and water
EHEC	Undercooked ground beef or beef, unpasteurized fruit juice, spinach
ETEC	Travel
EPEC	Infants in developing countries, nursery outbreaks
EAEC	Neonatal nursery outbreaks
Plesiomonas shigelloides	Raw shellfish, travel to Mexico
Salmonella	Beef; poultry; pork; eggs; dairy products; including unpasteurized milk; contaminated water; travel, bean sprouts; and other vegetables, contact with turtles, snakes, and other reptiles; chickens and other poultry
Shigella	Contaminated water and food, daycare exposure, travel
Vibrio cholera	Raw oysters, travel to endemic areas
Vibrio parahemolyticus	Raw shellfish and seafood consumption, foreign travel, travel to Louisiana and U.S. Gulf Coast region
Yersinia enterocolitica	Contaminated pork, chitterlings, tofu, unpasteurized milk
Viruses	Most viral causes of gastroenteritis are acquired through the oral–fecal route after direct contact with an infected person; in addition, Norwalk virus, rotavirus, and astroviruses can be acquired through contaminated water or food
Parasites	
Giardia lamblia	Contaminated water or food, contact with beavers, contact with infected individuals, poor sanitation, camping, travel
Cryptosporidium parvum	Contaminated water or food; contact with infected individuals or farm animals, particularly cows; travel
Cyclospora cayetenensis	Contaminated water or food, contact with infected individuals, travel
Entamoeba histolytica	Contaminated water or food, contact with infected individuals, travel

Pathogenic bacteria can be identified by isolating the organism by culture and/or by identifying a characteristic marker for virulence such as a toxin. Routine bacterial stool cultures can identify *Campylobacter, Salmonella, Shigella, Yersinia enterocolitica, Aeromonas hydrophila, Pleisiomonas shigelloides,* and noncholera *Vibrio* spp. Special media are required to identify *E. coli* O157:H7 and *Vibrio cholera,* and laboratory personnel should be notified when such agents are suspected. In addition to culture, *E. coli* O157:H7 can also be diagnosed using a toxin assay that detects shiga toxins produced by all EHEC types. Toxin assays rather than culture are routinely used for diagnosing *Clostridium difficile* diarrhea.

Because an outbreak was suspected from the school picnic our case patient attended, a stool culture was performed despite the fact that he had a mild self-limited illness. A routine bacterial stool culture would be appropriate in this case since *Salmonella, Shigella,* or *Campylobacter* spp. would be the most likely causes. His lack of bloody diarrhea would make EHEC, such as *E. coli* O157:H7, less likely. His lack of travel history indicates that his specimen does not need to be screened for organisms found outside his geographic area, and the absence of antibiotic use makes testing for toxins of *C. difficile* less of a priority.

Because there is no specific antiviral treatment available, testing for viral causes of gastroenteritis is not routinely performed except in outbreak situations or hospital settings. Testing for rotavirus, a major cause of fever, vomiting, and watery diarrhea in infants and young children, is routinely performed in hospitals so that patients can be cohorted and infection control practices emphasized. Rotavirus is commonly seen during the winter months (October–March).

Feces should be submitted in a clean, dry, plastic or waxed cardboard container with a tight-fitting or screwcap lid. Once collected, the specimen can be maintained at room temperature during transport. Rectal swabs should be used only with infants and young children from whom collecting feces may be difficult and again should be taken only during acute disease. For an adequate specimen, the swab should be inserted past the anal sphincter into the rectum, and feces should be obvious on the swab when removed. If the specimen (feces or swab) will not be processed or reach the laboratory within 1 h, an enteric transport medium should be inoculated with the feces and this will be stable for as long as 72 h at room temperature. In addition to stool, blood cultures should also be obtained from patients who have fever and diarrhea.

3.4. RESULTS

Stool specimens are different from other clinical specimens because of the large numbers and types of bacteria that constitute normal flora of the bowel. *Enterobacteriaceae,* nonfermenting gram-negative rods, staphylococci, enterococci, streptococci, yeast, and anaerobes are all considered normal fecal flora. The feces of normal adults contain between 10^{11} and 10^{12} bacteria per gram. The challenge for the laboratory is to isolate and identify from the vast fecal microflora those bacteria most likely to be implicated as causes of diarrhea. To achieve this goal, stool specimens are cultured

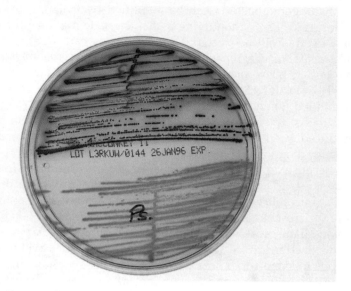

FIGURE 3.1 Lactose-fermenting colonies (top) and non-lactose-fermenting colonies (bottom) on MacConkey agar.

onto a battery of media that include two enteric media which are selective and differential for gram-negative rods, *Campylobacter* media that selects specifically for *Campylobacter* spp., and blood agar media. A medium that is "selective and differential" selects specifically for one group of organisms, in this case, gram-negative rods, and then differentiates between the types of gram-negative rods using either sugars such as lactose or bile salts. Different gram-negative rods can then be physically distinguished from each other by biochemical characteristics. For example, MacConkey agar is routinely used by many labs when culturing stool, and it allows for the growth of only gram-negative rods. Organisms that grow on MacConkey agar can then be differentiated from each other by their ability to ferment lactose. Lactose-fermenting gram-negative rods will be pink, and nonlactose fermenters will be clear (Fig. 3.1). Other enteric media contain H_2S indicators, which simplify the recognition of *Salmonella* spp. Most *Salmonella* produce H_2S, and as a result, the colonies appear black on the surface of the media (Fig. 3.2). Bloody stool specimens from patients suspected of having *E. coli* O157:H7 would also be inoculated onto sorbitol–MacConkey agar. *E. coli* O157:H7 are sorbitol-negative, and the colonies appear clear on the sorbitol–MacConkey media (Fig. 3.3). Following initial overnight incubation, media are carefully examined and any "suspicious" colonies are further tested biochemically to identify them. Once identified, *Salmonella* and *Shigella* spp. can be further grouped (groups A, B, C, etc.) using antisera. This is important information in outbreak situations.

After 24 h incubation, results of the stool culture from our case patient were reported as "Normal fecal flora with non-lactose-fermenting gram-negative rods." Both *Salmonella* and *Shigella* spp. appear as non-lactose-fermenting gram-negative rods on enteric media. This preliminary report indicates that the laboratory found suspicious colonies (because they were nonlactose fermenters). After 48 h, final results of the stool culture from

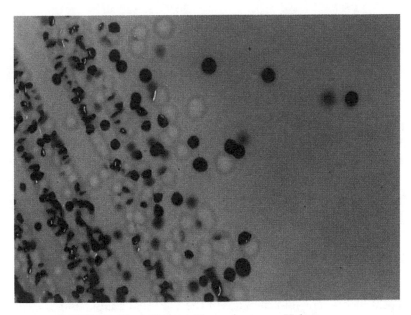

FIGURE 3.2 Black H$_2$S-positive colonies on Hektoen agar.

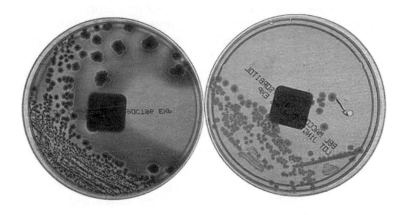

FIGURE 3.3 Sorbitol-positive (left) and sorbitol-negative (right) *E. coli.*

our case patient were reported as "Normal fecal flora and *Salmonella* spp, group B isolated." This indicated that *Salmonella* was identified from the sample and that when the O cell wall antigen was typed using specific agglutinating antisera, the isolate was further classified as group B. Antibiotic susceptibility test results showed our case patient's *Salmonella* isolate to be susceptible to ampicillin, ciprofloxacin, and trimethoprim–sulfamethoxazole (SXT). Of the 50 other students who became symptomatic after attending the school picnic, 34 had stool cultures positive for *Salmonella* spp., group B with antibiotic susceptibility results that matched those of the case patient. State public health authorities were notified of the results, and an epidemiologic investigation was initiated.

3.5. PATHOGENESIS

Enteric microorganisms cause gastrointestinal disease according to where and how they invade the GI tract. Some organisms stay in the lumen of the intestines and cause disease by forming a toxin or adhering to the cell surface, which prevents absorption of nutrients. With this type of infection, the patient presents with a watery diarrhea. With watery diarrhea there are a large volume and an increased number of stools, with an absence of fecal leukocytes. The patient has nausea and vomiting, cramping, abdominal pain, arthralgia, myalgia, and chills, but rarely any fever. Examples of this type of infection are those caused by ETEC or the parasite *Giardia lamblia*.

If the organism can invade the mucosa of the colon and distal small bowel, it causes an inflammatory colitis. The volume of stools passed is low, but the feces will contain numerous leukocytes, mucus, and blood (dysentery). The patient has fever, chills, cramping, and vomiting. Examples of bacteria that can invade the mucosa are EIEC, EHEC, *Shigella*, *Campylobacter*, and *Yersinia*. *Salmonella* are also invasive, but they do not produce mucosal ulcerations and damage in the way that EHEC and *Shigella* do. *Salmonella* invade the lamina propria of the small intestine and cause an inflammatory response at that site.

Some bacteria (*Salmonella typhi*, *Y. enterocolitica*) go one step further and penetrate deeper into the intestinal tissue and progress into the reticuloendothelial system (liver, spleen, bone marrow, and lymph nodes). From the lymph nodes *Salmonella* can enter the bloodstream, causing a disease called enteric fever. The patient has an acute illness of fever, headache, abdominal pain, splenomegaly, hepatomegaly, and rash on the upper abdomen and lower thorax called "rose spots." *S. typhi* and *S. paratyphi* cause an illness known as typhoid fever, because the patient initially presents with a systemic illness (fever, malaise, rash) rather than a diarrheal disease; in fact, patients are often constipated in the early weeks of illness. Because most patients with typhoid fever develop bacteremia, blood cultures should be performed when *S. typhi* is suspected. Later in the illness (≥3 weeks) the patient has diarrhea and the organism can be cultured from the stool. Nontyphoid *Salmonella* are associated with a much lower rate of bacteremia, so routine blood cultures are not recommended except in special patient groups, such as infants and young children or those with sickle cell disease or human immunodeficiency virus (HIV).

Y. enterocolitica also disseminates into the mesenteric lymph nodes and causes lower quadrant pain and fever. The presentation mimics acute appendicitis, and some patients have even undergone surgery, only to discover a normal appendix when the histopathology is reviewed.

The organisms causing gastroenteritis or enteric fever demonstrate a variety of pathogenic mechanisms and virulence factors. A battery of toxins and invasive mechanisms result in watery diarrhea, dysentery, or enteric fever. Organisms with more than one mechanism of pathogenesis, such as *Campylobacter* spp., may present with more than one type of diarrheal syndrome. The clinically important bacteria that cause acute diarrhea in humans are listed in Table 3.2 along with the type of diarrhea they cause and the virulence factors they possess.

TABLE 3.2. **Types of Diarrhea Caused by Bacterial Pathogens and Their Mechanisms of Pathogenesis**

Organism	Type of Diarrhea	Mechanism of Pathogenesis
Campylobacter jejuni/coli	Watery	Cholera-like enterotoxin
	Dysentery	Cytotoxins
		Organism uses chemotaxis and flagellum to colonize mucus in distal ileum and colon; motility also a virulence factor
Salmonella spp.	Watery	Enterotoxin activates cAMP
	Dysentery	Cytotoxin inhibits protein synthesis
		Organism produces adhesion that stimulates rearrangement of host cell membrane, "ruffles," which engulf the bacteria into cell; bacteria invade large and small bowel and lamina propria
Salmonella typhi, S. paratyphi A, B, C	Enteric fever (typhoid fever)	Organism invades mucosa; multiplies in liver, spleen, and lymphoid tissue; escapes into bloodstream via macrophages, which do not kill the bacteria
Shigella spp.	Dysentery	Cytotoxin/verotoxin/shigatoxin
		Organism enters cells by phagocytic vacuole, then escapes into the cytoplasm; an actin "tail" propels bacteria into new cells
Clostridium difficile	Watery	Enterotoxin A causes fluid accumulation
	Dysentery	Cytotoxin B causes cell death
Yersinia enterocolitica	Dysentery; enteric fever-like	Invades mucosa
Vibrio parahaemolyticus	Watery	Shiga-like toxins
		Thermostable direct hemolysin
Vibrio cholera	Watery	Two-part enterotoxin: B subunit binds toxin to host cell, A subunit activates cAMP, causing hypersecretion of Na^+, K^+, HCO_3^- ions resulting in fluid accumulation in intestinal lumen, leading to dehydrating diarrhea without damage to mucosa
Enterotoxigenic *E. coli* (ETEC)	Watery	Colonization factor antigen pili allow colonization of small bowel; two toxins produced—heat-labile toxin (LT) = cholera-like toxin, heat-stable toxin (ST)
Enterohemorrhagic *E. coli* (EHEC)	Dysentery	Cytotoxin or shiga-like toxin acting on rRNA to block protein synthesis, causing cell death
Enteropathogenic *E. coli* (EPEC)	Watery	Mediated by bundle-forming pili, organism aggregates onto microvilli and produces attaching and effacing lesions
Enteroinvasive *E. coli* (EIEC)	Dysentery	Organism invades large bowel, causing ulceration, inflammation, necrosis

TABLE 3.2.	Types of Diarrhea Caused by Bacterial Pathogens and Their Mechanisms of Pathogenesis	
Organism	Type of Diarrhea	Mechanism of Pathogenesis
Enteroaggregative E. coli (EAEC)	Watery	Organism adheres to mucosa like "stacked bricks" and prevents absorption by microvilli
Aeromonas hydrophila	Watery Dysentery	Bundle-forming pili act as intestinal colonization factors Hemolysins Enterotoxin
Plesiomonas shigelloides	Watery Dysentery	Unknown—suspected to be toxigenic and invasive

Patients with gastroenteritis acquire their infections by ingesting contaminated food or drink. Animals may carry *Salmonella* or EHEC strains as part of their normal flora, and improper handling and cooking of these food products can lead to infection. Petting animals, such as calves at a "petting zoo," can be sufficient exposure to *Salmonella* to transmit the bacteria and cause disease.

Shigella is the exception since there are no animal reservoirs for these bacteria. Transmission is always fecal–oral from one person to another or contaminated water. Unlike *Salmonella*, which requires 10,000 organisms, relatively few organisms of *Shigella* (between 10 and 100) can cause disease. Once *Shigella* infects a person, the bacteria can be easily transmitted from person to person, unless good hand-washing practices are used.

3.6. TREATMENT AND PREVENTION

The first line of therapy is supportive treatment, to return the patient to fluid and electrolyte balance. The patient may drink an oral rehydration solution that contains water, salt, and sugar, or liquids such as Pedialyte, which have the appropriate electrolytes and fluids to replace those being lost. Most cases of gastroenteritis are self-limited and require no antibiotic therapy. In fact, antibiotics are contraindicated in some cases. Giving antibiotics for *Salmonella* gastroenteritis prolongs the carriage of the organism in the GI tract and can lead to the person retaining the organism for months. Treatment of *E. coli* O157:H7 may increase the risk of hemolytic uremic syndrome (HUS) in children and should be avoided. Likewise, one should avoid using antimotility agents in cases with bloody diarrhea or proven EHEC infection.

Patients who are very young or immunosuppressed may require antibiotics to recover from their disease. Patients with *Shigella* gastroenteritis are more likely to be sicker and require antibiotic therapy than are patients with *Salmonella* or *Campylobacter* gastroenteritis.

Ampicillin, SXT, or ciprofloxacin are common choices for antimicrobial therapy because they can be administered orally if the patient can tolerate drinking liquids. Since the organism may be resistant to one or more of these antimicrobials, susceptibility results for the patient's organism should guide the physician's choice.

According to surveillance by the Centers for Disease Control and Prevention (CDC), *Campylobacter jejuni* is the most common enteric pathogen seen in adult patients with diarrhea, whereas *Salmonella* is the most common in children. *Campylobacter* spp. are not susceptible to penicillins or cephalosporins. Ciprofloxacin and erythromycin are the drugs of choice.

If a patient is hospitalized with enteric fever (*S. typhi*), a third-generation cephalosporin is usually given intravenously. Our case patient has an infection with *Salmonella* susceptible to ampicillin, SXT, and ciprofloxacin. Because he is a healthy young adult, only supportive treatment was given.

3.7. ADDITIONAL POINTS

- If multiple bacterial cultures are not diagnostic and the patient continues to have symptoms, examination of the stool for ova and parasites is the next step. At least three stool specimens collected on three separate days may be required to detect a parasitic infection since parasites are shed intermittently.

- Most laboratories will not perform Gram stains of fecal material because enteric pathogens cannot be differentiated from normal fecal flora on Gram stain; however, the presence of WBCs may be indicative of an invasive pathogen.

- Patients with sickle cell disease are more likely to acquire *Salmonella* infections that enter the bloodstream during their acute diarrhea. This is because their macrophages are already overextended in cleaning up red cell debris from the sickle cell disease and cannot fight the *Salmonella* infection and contain it to the GI tract.

- When *Salmonella* disseminates, it often goes to the long bones and causes an infection of the bone (osteomyelitis). Radiographic changes are visible, and the organism can be cultured from blood. Infants and young children are more susceptible to developing osteomyelitis as a result of *Salmonella* bacteremia.

- Carriers of *Salmonella* are those who continue to shed the bacteria in the stool more than 6 months after the initial infection. The organism can reside in the gallbladder, and low numbers of *Salmonella* are shed in the stool. The patients are asymptomatic, but they can transmit the bacteria to others when preparing food. Food handlers are usually screened with a stool culture before employment to detect the carrier state. For those who are entering an institution, stool screening is a normal procedure to prevent transmission among residents.

- In normal hosts, gastric acid destroys many pathogenic enteric bacteria and is an important host factor in resisting diarrheal infections. People who routinely consume large amounts of antacids or bicarbonate and thus change the pH levels of the stomachs will increase their risk of acquiring enteric infections.

■ Culturing food products is not done routinely in a hospital laboratory. If contaminated food is suspected, all products in their original containers should be taken to the state public health laboratory for further investigation.

■ An acute paralytic disease of the peripheral nervous system (Guillain–Barré syndrome) is associated with a preceding infection of *Campylobacter jejuni*. It is proposed that lipopolysaccharide antigens of the *Campylobacter* cross-react with peripheral nerve tissue and that the cellular response by the host leads to nerve cell damage.

■ *C. difficile* is the most likely cause of diarrhea in patients whose symptoms develop after ≥3 days of hospitalization. It is highly unlikely that they are eating food products contaminated with *Salmonella*, *Shigella*, or *Campylobacter*. A stool sample should be submitted to detect the presence of toxins A and B to confirm the diagnosis. Since these toxins are unstable after the stool is collected, the specimen must be transported to the lab immediately or refrigerated until such transport is possible. *C. difficile*–associated diarrhea (CDAD) may progress to pseudomembranous colitis, and severe symptoms that may require surgical intervention. Taking antibiotics that wipe out the normal bowel flora is a risk factor for acquiring CDAD. Stopping the offending antibiotic, treating the *C. difficile* with oral vancomycin or metroniazole, isolating the patient, and utilizing excellent hand hygiene and environmental disinfection are required to control the disease and prevent the transmission of the infection.

SUGGESTED READING

DENNEHY, P. H., Acute diarrheal disease in children: Epidemiology, prevention, and treatment, *Infect. Dis. Clin. N. Am.* **19**: 585–602 (2005).

DuPONT, H. L., What's new in enteric infectious diseases at home and abroad, *Curr. Opin. Infect. Dis.* **18**: 407–412 (2005).

GUERRANT, R. L., T. VAN GILDER, T. S. STEINER ET AL., Practice guidelines for the management of infectious diarrhea, *Clin. Infect. Dis.* **32**: 331–350 (2001).

WELINDER-OLSSON, C. AND B. KAIJSER, Enterohemorrhagic *Escherichia coli* (EHEC), *Scand. J. Infect. Dis.* **37**: 405–416 (2005).

Chronic Diarrhea in a Traveler

4.1. PATIENT HISTORY

A 21 year-old male presents with a 6-week history of watery diarrhea and crampy abdominal pain. He reports that the diarrhea has not been constant and has alternated with periods of constipation. For the past 2 weeks, the diarrhea has been blood-streaked and he has had several weeks of midepigastric pain. He spent the past 6 months in a rural community in Guatemala participating in a community service project sponsored by his college. He returned from Guatemala just 10 days ago. While there, he drank the water and ate the food available in the local community, and he did not routinely boil water for drinking. He denies antibiotic exposure but has taken mefloquine weekly for malaria prophylaxis. Two separate stool specimens taken by student health when he returned were reported as negative for *Salmonella*, *Shigella*, *Campylobacter*, *E. coli O157:H7*, *Yersinia*, *Aeromonas*, and *Pleisiomonas* as well as *Giardia lamblia*. On physical examination he appeared well nourished and well developed but reports an 8–10 lb weight loss. He was afebrile with a blood pressure of 110/80 mm Hg, pulse rate of 84/min, and respirations of 14/min, and his lungs were clear. The abdominal examination was significant for tenderness localized to the right upper quadrant without rebound tenderness, but no mass or hepatomegaly was appreciated.

Medical Microbiology for the New Curriculum: A Case-Based Approach, by Roberta B. Carey, Mindy G. Schuster, and Karin L. McGowan.

4.2. DIFFERENTIAL DIAGNOSIS

"Traveler's diarrhea" is loose, watery diarrhea that occurs within the first week of arriving in a new country. The diarrhea is usually accompanied by nausea, vomiting, abdominal cramps, and fever; however, the disease is self-limited, and the average length of illness is 3–5 days. The risk of acquiring traveler's diarrhea increases in less-developed countries and the disease is transmitted via fecally contaminated food or water.

Infectious Causes

Organisms responsible for causing traveler's diarrhea include those listed below.

Bacteria

Aeromonas spp.

Campylobacter spp.

Enterotoxigenic E. coli (ETEC), accounting for 50% of cases

Plesiomonas shigelloides

Salmonella spp.

Shigella spp.

Vibrio spp.

Viruses

Rotavirus

Calcivirus (Norwalk)

Parasites

Cryptosporidium parvum

Cyclospora cayetenensis

Entamoeba histolytica

Giardia lamblia

Isospora belli

Fungi and Mycobacteria

There are no agents in these categories that routinely cause traveler's diarrhea in a normal host.

Discussion

Because his symptoms have persisted for 6 weeks, this patient is unlikely to have traveler's diarrhea. The length of his illness fulfills the criteria for chronic ($\geq$3 weeks) diarrhea. This patient also has significant findings on abdominal exam, and if a liver abscess was also present, the differential would expand to include a bacterial or parasitic abscess of the liver and liver cancer. The differential for chronic diarrhea and liver abscesses in a normal host would include parasitic infections, abdominal abscess, and noninfectious causes.

Other Infectious Causes

Bacteria Likely to Cause Abdominal or Liver Abscesses
These would include:

Anaerobes

Enteric gram-negative rods (*Escherichia coli, Klebsiella* spp., *Enterobacter* spp.)

Staphylococcus spp.

Streptococcus spp.

Parasites Associated with Chronic Diarrhea
These would include:

Cryptosporidium parvum

Cyclospora cayetenensis

Echinococcus granulosus—also associated with liver abscess

Entamoeba histolytica—also associated with liver abscess

Isospora belli

Viruses, Fungi and Mycobacteria
There are no agents in these categories that routinely cause chronic diarrhea in a normal host.

Noninfectious Causes

Ulcerative colitis

Inflammatory bowel disease

Crohn's disease

Diverticulitis

Carcinoma

CLINICAL CLUES

? Have the symptoms persisted for more than a week? Think chronic causes of diarrhea such as parasites.

? Has the patient drunk well water, water from streams, or nonpotable water? Think parasites such as *Giardia, Cryptosporidium*, or *Cyclospora*.

? Are routine bacterial cultures of stool negative? Check which pathogens were looked for, think of less commonly seen *Vibrio, Yersinia*, viruses, or parasites.

4.3. LABORATORY TESTS

Just as with acute diarrhea, the history of a patient's illness frequently provides clues to the etiology of the disease. The length of illness and travel history of this patient plus abdominal findings and weight loss are key features. Diarrhea with blood narrows infectious causes to agents such as *Shigella*, *Salmonella*, *Campylobacter*, EHEC, EIEC, and *Entamoeba histolytica*. An evaluation for chronic diarrhea requires a stool culture (×3), ova and parasite exam of stool (×3), and guaiac test of stool for occult blood. Because of this patient's abdominal findings, liver function tests such as alkaline phosphatase and serum transaminases should also be ordered. Whenever liver abscess is suspected, abdominal ultrasound or computed tomography (CT scan) should also be performed.

Because both bacteria and parasites can be shed intermittently in stool, multiple stool specimens should be submitted for both bacterial culture and ova and parasite examination. See Case 3 for information on stool collection and transport for bacterial culture. For parasite analysis, specimens should be taken on separate days (every other day if possible) to increase likelihood of detection. Stool specimens collected for parasite analysis should be submitted in preservation vial(s) designed for this purpose (Fig. 4.1). All forms of parasites (ova, larvae, protozoa, worms) can be maintained at room temperature for long periods of time (months) using preservation vials. In addition, concentration procedures to recover small numbers of protozoan cysts, eggs, and larvae can be performed using the vials, and permanent stained smears can be prepared as well. If preservation vials are not available, then stool should be collected in clean, dry,

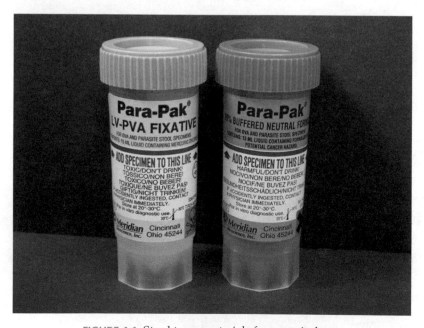

FIGURE 4.1 Stool transport vials for parasitology.

wide-mouthed containers with tight-fitting lids. The stool should not be contaminated with urine because the pH of urine can destroy motile parasites. Liquid stool specimens must be examined by the laboratory within 30 min after they were taken from the patient, or some parasitic forms will disintegrate. If this rapid transport time is not possible, then preservation vials should be used.

Results of an initial ova and parasite stool examination showed that the specimen was positive for cysts of *E. histolytica/E. dispar*. With this additional information, a serology test for *E. histolytica* antibodies and an abdominal CT scan were ordered.

E. histolytica, the cause of intestinal amebiasis and amebic liver abscess, can be diagnosed in the laboratory using a variety of methods:

1. *Microscopic exam (stool, liver abscess)*. Microscopic identification of *E. histolytica* cysts or trophozoite (ameboid) forms is the most common method used to diagnose the infection; however, it is both insensitive and nonspecific. The test is nonspecific because *E. histolytica* cysts cannot be morphologically distinguished from those of *Entamoeba dispar*, a harmless commensal, unless ingested RBCs are present inside the trophozoite. Microscopic examination of liver abscess material is a poor way to attempt the diagnosis of amebiasis. While the abscess material is known to have the appearance of "anchovy paste," ameba are rarely visualized in the material because they have disintegrated.

2. *Antibody detection (serum)*. Serology studies [indirect hemagglutination, gel diffusion, enzyme-linked immunosorbent assay (ELISA)] to detect antibody to *E. histolytica* are positive in >90% of patients who have invasive disease. In the vast majority of patients antibodies are detectable after 7–10 days. When patients no longer have detectable parasites in their stools, detection of antibodies is critical for diagnosis of amebic liver abscesses.

3. *Antigen detection (stool)*. Detection of antigen from stool is an extremely sensitive and specific method to diagnose *E. histolytica*. Stool antigen kits are commercially available, and the test can be performed in 2 h. Antigen detection testing requires the use of fresh or frozen (not preserved) stool. Despite the superb sensitivity of this test, the number of patients seen in a routine clinical setting in the United States (nonendemic area) may be too small to support this test in a routine hospital laboratory. When needed, this test can be sent to a reference lab.

4. *Colonoscopy*. Biopsy specimens or aspirated material from colonic lesions can be microscopically examined for ameba of *E. histolytica*. Wet preparations of material aspirated or scraped from the ulcers should be examined immediately for motile ameba. Biopsy material, which should be taken from the outer edge of the ulcer, can be stained to visualize amebic forms.

5. *Polymerase chain reaction (PCR)*. PCR assays of stool, culture of stool or liver abscess, and isoenzyme analysis are largely research tools at this time and for a variety of reasons are not practical tests for hospital laboratories to perform.

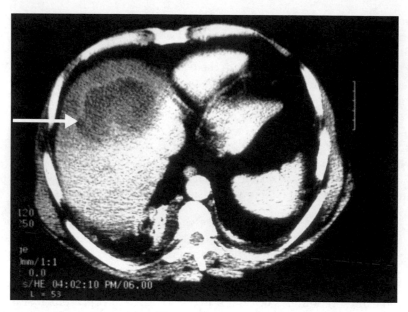

FIGURE 4.2 CT scan showing liver abscess.

4.4. RESULTS

The following laboratory results were available on our patient after 72 h:

Alkaline phosphatase = 200 U/L (elevated)

Aspartate aminotransferase = 35 U/L (normal)

Alanine aminotransferase = 42 U/L (normal)

Guaiac test = negative

Stool cultures = negative for *Salmonella, Shigella, Campylobacter*, EHEC

Ova and parasite exams = positive for cysts of *E. histolytica/E. dispar*

Serology = positive titer for *E. histolytica* IgG of 1: 2048 (normal titer ≤ 1: 128)

The abdominal CT scan revealed a 10-cm, irregular cystic mass on the posterior wall of the right lobe of the liver (Fig. 4.2). Abdominal ultrasound or CT scan is equally sensitive at detecting abscesses, but neither of the two techniques can actually differentiate an amebic abscess from a bacterial abscess. A positive IgG antibody titer to *E. histolytica* confirmed the CT finding as an amebic abscess. The definitive diagnosis of amebic liver abscess is made by a positive serology plus the demonstration of a hepatic abscess (Fig. 4.3).

4.5. PATHOGENESIS

Humans serve as the major reservoir of *E. histolytica* infections. Although infections occur worldwide, there is a higher incidence in those living in

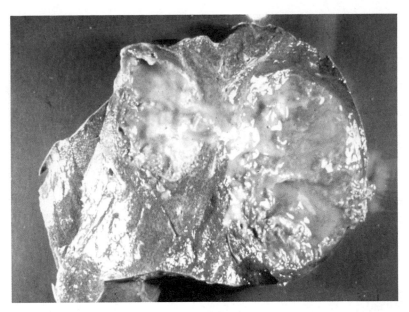

FIGURE 4.3 *Entamoeba histolytica* liver abscess on gross exam.

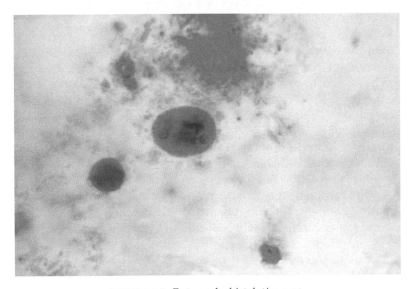

FIGURE 4.4 *Entamoeba histolytica* cyst.

the tropics. Only 10% of those infected with *E. histolytica* have clinical symptoms, and 90% are asymptomatic carriers, who shed the cysts in their stools and transmit the infection to others. *E. histolytica* occurs in two forms: the cyst that contains four nuclei and is 9–19 μm in diameter (Fig. 4.4) and the ameboid trophozoite that possesses one nucleus and is 12–60 μm long (Fig. 4.5). The trophozoite is the motile form that lives in the large intestine, reproduces under anaerobic conditions, and causes tissue damage. The cyst is the infectious form. Resistant to gastric acid, the cyst is excreted into the stool and may be ingested by a new host in contaminated

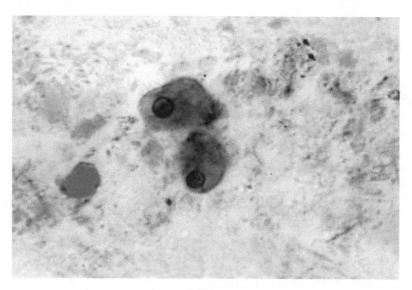

FIGURE 4.5 *Entamoeba histolytica* trophozoites.

food or water. Hyperchlorination or iodination of the water will destroy the infectious cysts.

In the large intestine, cysts mature into trophozoites, which can break down the mucosal barrier of the colon with proteinases. The parasite then adheres to the target cell using a galactose-*N*-acetyl-*O*-galactosamine adhesion lectin. Channel forming peptides (amebapores) transport nutrients to the trophozoites and exert cytolytic activity. Rapid cytolytic changes occur that kill target cells, polymorphonuclear leukocytes, and macrophages. The parasite remains unharmed and continues to invade tissue by locomotion, attachment, and adhesion. Proteolytic degradation of the extracellular matrix of the colon results in tissue necrosis.

Trophozoites of *E. histolytica* produce a focal ulceration of the colonic mucosa that can present as colicky pain and bloody diarrhea (dysentery), fulminating colitis, or amebic appendicitis. Ulceration of the infected mucosa occurs at several sites with normal mucosa between the ulcers. The ulcers deepen and form a classic flask-shaped ulcer of amebic colitis that extends to the mucosa and muscularis mucosa into the submucosa (Fig. 4.6). These ulcers can be infected secondarily with bacteria. Chronic ulceration can lead to the formation of a palpable mass of granulation tissue, called an ameboma, which can mimic a malignant tumor in the cecum, colon, or rectum. Perforation of the colon by the amebic ulcer occurs in 21% of patients and may result in peritonitis and dissemination to the liver, lungs, pericardium, brain, and skin. A liver abscess in the right upper lobe is the most common extraintestinal form of invasive amebiasis.

Patients with a liver abscess may have no history of *E. histolytica*. They present with right upper quadrant pain, fever, leukocytosis without eosinophilia (eosinophils increase in most extraintestinal parasitic infections), elevated alkaline phosphatase and transaminase levels, and a high erythrocyte sedimentation rate. A cardinal sign of liver abscess is painful hepatomegaly. Liver abscesses occur more frequently in adults than in

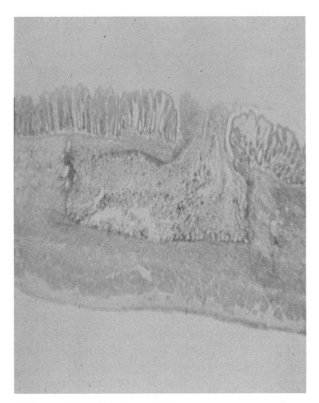

FIGURE 4.6 Flask-shaped ulcer of *E. histolytica.*

children and more frequently in males. The contents of the liver abscess are described as "anchovy paste" because of the chocolate brown color of the material, which is usually sterile for bacteria. Serology tests are positive in 75% of patients with intestinal amebiasis and in 90% of patients with liver abscesses, but a negative serology test does not rule out the possibility of an amebic infection.

Risk groups for *E. histolytica* infection include travelers to developing countries, immigrants, migrant workers, immunocompromised patients, and homosexuals. *E. histolytica* is one of the major pathogens causing "gay bowel syndrome" in homosexuals. Direct oral–anal contact leads to fecal exposure and oral contact with a variety of intestinal parasites.

Other parasitic ameba exist in nature but are not considered pathogenic for humans. To distinguish *E. histolytica* from the nonpathogenic *Entamoeba coli* and other ameba, careful attention to the characteristics of the nuclei is mandatory. *E. histolytica* have delicate chromatin in the nuclear membrane and a small compact karyosome in the center of the nucleus. Humans are infected by two morphologically identical species of *Entamoeba*: *E. histolytica*, that causes amebic colitis and liver abscesses; and *E. dispar*, which is noninvasive. On routine microscopic examination, the laboratory cannot tell the difference between them. Pathogenic *E. histolytica* can be differentiated from the commensal parasite, *E. dispar*, by electrophoretic separation of isoenyzmes (zymodeme analysis), specific antigen detection tests, or by PCR.

4.6. TREATMENT AND PREVENTION

Two classes of drugs are used to treat *E. histolytica* infections. (1) a luminal amebicide, such as iodoquinol, which destroys parasites in the lumen of the intestine but does not kill ameba in tissue; and (2) a tissue amebicide, such as metronidazole or chloroquine, which treats invasive amebiasis but is less effective in the lumen. Amebic dysentery may be treated with iodoquinol and metronidazole. Extraintestinal disease is treated with a combination of metronidazole and chloroquine. To follow the clinical response of intestinal disease to therapy, a repeat stool exam for parasites should be done 2–4 weeks after treatment, and extraintestinal disease should be monitored by repeat CT scans. Repeat serology tests are of little use since antibody titers remain elevated in spite of response to therapy. Prevention of infection with *E. histolytica* involves drinking boiled or bottled water when traveling to developing nations, and avoiding uncooked foods that may have been washed in water, such as salad.

4.7. ADDITIONAL POINTS

■ The list of infectious agents causing chronic diarrhea expands considerably in patients with AIDS to include opportunistic pathogens. It would include parasites such as *Cryptosporidium* spp., *Cyclospora* spp., *Isospora* spp., and microsporidia (*Enterocytozoon*, *Encephalitozoon*), as well as *Mycobacterium avium-intracellulare* (MAI) and cytomegalovirus.

■ *Cryptosporidium, Cyclospora*, and *Isospora* may be difficult to detect on routine microscopic exam. Their microscopic detection is enhanced with a modified acid-fast stain, which stains these parasites pink to red. These parasites are distinguished from one another by careful measurement of the size of the cysts and noting their characteristic shape microscopically (Fig. 4.7). A modified acid-fast stain to detect these parasites and a

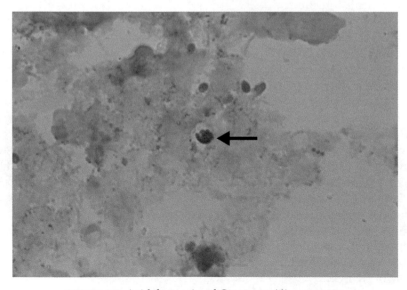

FIGURE 4.7 Acid-fast stain of *Cryptosporidium parvum.*

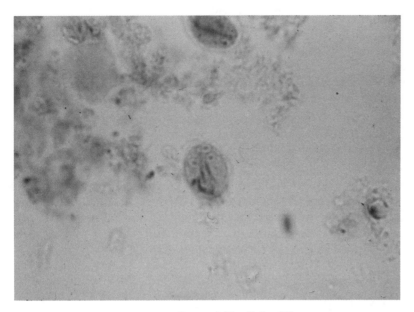

FIGURE 4.8 Cysts of *Giardia lamblia.*

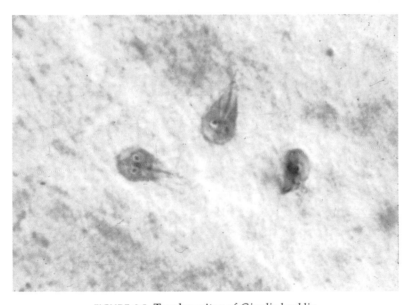

FIGURE 4.9 Trophozoites of *Giardia lamblia.*

special stain to detect microsporidia should be ordered when diagnosing persistent diarrhea in AIDS patients.

■ *Giardia lamblia* is the most common parasitic infection in the United States. It is the most common cause of chronic diarrhea in travelers (Figs. 4.8, 4.9). Unlike *E. histolytica*, which is invasive, *G. lamblia* causes a watery diarrhea by covering the brushed border of the small intestine, resulting in atrophy of the microvilli and villi, malabsorption of electrolytes and enzyme deficiencies.

■ At some centers, abdominal ultrasound is preferred over CT scan to diagnose an amebic abscess because the ultrasound can be performed more rapidly, at less cost, and with less toxicity, and can differentiate biliary disease from hepatic disease. CT scan, however, is thought to be more sensitive in the detection of small abscesses and to provide greater resolution.

■ Aspiration of a liver abscess may be done to rule out a bacterial abscess, to reduce the risk of liver rupture, or to treat the patient if there has been no response to medical treatment after 72 h.

■ Most cases of diarrhea in travelers are self-limited if the host is immunocompetent. In children, however, the disease can be fatal because of severe depletion of their electrolytes. For adults the disease is responsible for lost time at work and thus has economic consequences. In the immunocompromised patient, infection and diarrhea may persist with little clinical response to appropriate therapy.

SUGGESTED READING

AYEH-KUNI, P. F., M. PHIL, AND W.A. PETRI, Diagnosis and management of amebiasis, *Infect. Med.* **19**: 375–382 (2002).

DIEMERT, D. J., Prevention and self-treatment of traveler's diarrhea, *Clin. Microbiol. Rev.* **19**: 583–594 (2006).

DUPONT, H. L., What's new in enteric infectious diseases at home and abroad, *Curr. Opin. Infect. Dis.* **18**: 407–412 (2005).

ESPINOSA-CANTELLANO, M. AND A. MARTINEZ-PALOMO, Pathogenesis of intestinal amebiasis: From molecules to disease, *Clin. Microbiol. Rev.* **13**: 318–331 (2000).

OKHUYSEN, P. C., Current concepts in traveler's diarrhea: Epidemiology, antimicrobial resistance and treatment, *Curr. Opin. Infect. Dis.* **18**: 522–526 (2005).

Boy with Skin Lesions

5.1. PATIENT HISTORY

A 5 year-old boy presented to his pediatrician with a 3-week complaint of mildly itchy, scaly patches, particularly on his arms and back. Physical exam (PE) revealed a happy, alert child in no apparent distress, and review of systems was unremarkable except for cutaneous lesions. More than a dozen raised, red, scaling lesions were observed on his back; several had pinpoint pustules on the edges, and others had grown together to form larger polycyclic lesions. On his arms, a number of oval or ring-shaped lesions were present with redness and scaling (Fig. 5.1). All of the lesions were clear in the center. Of note, the family lives in a rural area and has many pets, including two dogs, three cats, and a ferret, and the boy plays with and participates in the care of all the animals. A potassium hydroxide (KOH) preparation of skin scrapings was performed in the office and was negative; however, additional skin scraping specimens were taken and submitted to the laboratory.

5.2. DIFFERENTIAL DIAGNOSIS

Skin rashes in infants and young children are quite common, and few are serious. The absence of fever in this boy's history and physical exam narrows the choices for differential diagnosis considerably. Many systemic illnesses (rickettsial, meningococcemia, etc.) are accompanied by a

Medical Microbiology for the New Curriculum: A Case-Based Approach, by Roberta B. Carey, Mindy G. Schuster, and Karin L. McGowan.

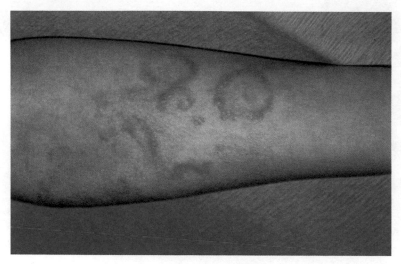

FIGURE 5.1 Skin lesion.

characteristic rash; however, most have significant fever as well. This patient's illness appears to be strictly cutaneous (itch and skin lesions) not systemic in nature.

Infectious Causes

Bacteria

Arcanobacterium haemolyticum

Borrelia burgdorferi (Lyme disease—erythema migrans)

Staphylococcus aureus

Streptococcus pyogenes (group A streptococcus)

Treponema pallidum

Viruses

Human herpesvirus 6 and 7 (HHV-6 and HHV-7)

Measles virus

Molluscipox virus (*Molluscum contagiosum*)

Parvovirus B19 (Fifth disease)

Fungi

Candida spp.

Dermatophytes: *Epidermophyton* spp., *Microsporum* spp., *Trichophyton* spp.

Malassezia furfur

Parasites

Ancylostoma spp. (cutaneous larva migrans)

Pediculus humanus corporis (body lice)

Sarcoptes scabei (scabies)

Noninfectious Causes

Contact dermatitis

Granuloma annulare

Mycoses fungoides (cutaneous T-cell lymphoma)

Nummular eczema

Pityriasis rosea

Psoriasis

CLINICAL CLUES

? Red, circular patches on the skin without ulceration in a healthy patient? Think dermatophyte, eczema, or contact dermatitis.

? Skin lesions in a patient with animals in the household? Think dermatophyte or parasite.

? Patches of alopecia (baldness) with hair broken off close to the scalp so that it looks like black dots? Think dermatophyte infection.

5.3. LABORATORY TESTS

Skin scrapings obtained from this patient were sent to the laboratory for both bacterial and fungal cultures. The area should be disinfected using alcohol-soaked gauze and then skin lesions should be scraped using a sterile scalpel blade. The centers of the skin rings or patches are frequently nonviable, so when collecting skin specimens, the outer actively growing margin of the lesion should be sampled. This is often called the "leading edge" of a skin lesion. With children, sterile toothbrushes are used to sample both skin and hair by vigorously brushing over the infected area. The entire brush should be sent to the laboratory. When it is not practical to scrape an area because the site is wet or oozing, a swab may be used. When examining the skin lesions on this child, a ringworm infection was strongly suspected. Despite its name, "ringworm" is not a worm but rather a fungal infection. Ringworm is the common name for an infection caused by a group of moulds called dermatophytes. These fungi grow in areas of the body that contain keratin, namely, hair, skin, and nails (Table 5.1). Three genera of organisms are classified as dermatophytes: *Trichophyton* spp., *Microsporum* spp., and *Epidermophyton floccosum*.

TABLE 5.1. **Areas Where Dermatophytes May Cause Infection**

Genus	Areas Infected
Microsporum	Hair and skin
Epidermophyton	Skin and nails
Trichophyton	Hair, skin, and nails

TABLE 5.2.	Names for Dermatophyte Infections Based on Body Site Infected	
Body Site	Medical Name	Common Name
Beard	Tinea barbae	Ringworm of the beard
Body/skin	Tinea corporis	Ringworm of the body
Feet	Tinea pedis	Athelete's foot
Genital area	Tinea cruris	"Jock" itch
Hand	Tinea manuum	Ringworm of the hand
Nail (finger/toe)	Tinea unguium, or onychomycosis	Ringworm of the nail
Scalp	Tinea capitis	Fungal infection/ringworm of the scalp or skin around eyebrows or eyelashes

The word 'tinea' means ring, and it has been used to clinically describe the skin lesions seen. Traditionally, dermatophyte infections have been named according to their anatomic location by appending the Latin name for the body site after the word tinea. Examples of this nomenclature are listed in Table 5.2.

For infected hair, the basal root is the best portion to use for microscopy and/or culture. For this reason, plucking some of the infected hairs to obtain the root is recommended. When examining affected hair, a Wood's light may be used to visualize the infected hairs. A Wood's light emits short wave (320–400 nm) UV radiation, also called "black light." Some dermatophytes produce characteristic fluorescence under UV light because they produce the chemical pteridine. Members of the *Microsporum* genus emit a blue-green or yellow fluorescence; the yeast *Malassezia furfur* emits a yellowish-white or copper-orange fluorescence. *E. floccosum* and most *Trichophyton* species with the exception of *T. schoenleinii* (dull yellow) are nonfluorescent.

The easiest method used to confirm the diagnosis of ringworm is with a 20–25% potassium hydroxide (KOH) test. To perform the test, hair or skin specimens are obtained and a portion of this material is placed on a glass slide with several drops of 20% KOH. The mixture is then heated, or dimethyl sulfoxide may be added so that heating is not necessary. The KOH creates single layers of epithelial cells, allowing hyphae, spores, or yeast cells that were trapped in the matrix to be visible by 400× magnification light microscopy (Fig. 5.2). The calcofluor white technique can also be used, but because it requires fluorescent microscopy, in contrast to the KOH prep, it is not suitable for a physician's office (Fig. 5.3). Because direct microscopy is falsely negative 15–20% of the time, culture should also be performed. When culturing for dermatophytes, culture media supplemented with cyclohexamide and chloramphenicol are used to inhibit the growth of bacteria and nondermatophyte moulds. Mycobiotic and mycosel agars are the most frequently used. Dermatophyte species tend to grow surrounded by agar medium rather than on top of the medium. For

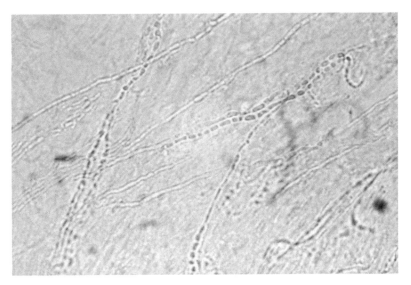

FIGURE 5.2 Positive KOH preparation.

this reason, when specimens are submitted on toothbrushes, the brushes should be lightly pressed into the medium in three or four places to inoculate the plate (Fig. 5.4). Nail sections should be pressed to submerge them just under the plate surface. Most dermatophytes take 2–5 days to grow on culture media (aerobic, room temperature), and isolates are identified to genus and species by their colony color and texture (Fig. 5.5), microscopic appearance (Fig. 5.3, 5.6), (Table 5.3), and reaction to specific physiological tests.

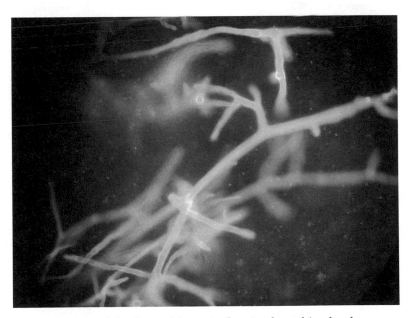

FIGURE 5.3 Calcofluor white stain showing branching hyphae.

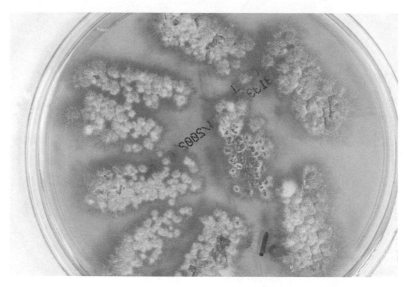

FIGURE 5.4 Mould on mycosel agar following inoculation with toothbrush.

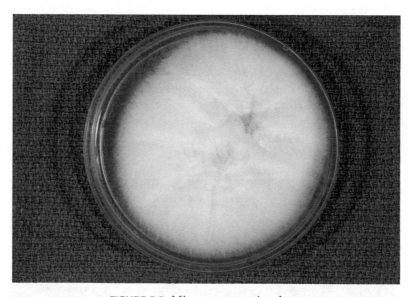

FIGURE 5.5 *Microsporum canis* colony

TABLE 5.3.	Comparison of Microscopic Features of Dermatophytes
Genus	Microscopic Features
Microsporum spp.	Abundant macroconidia that have spines on thick cell wall, with very few microconidia
Epidermophyton sp.	Macroconidia only, seen in bunches; thick cell wall
Trichophyton spp.	Abundant microconidia, few macroconidia, which are smooth-walled

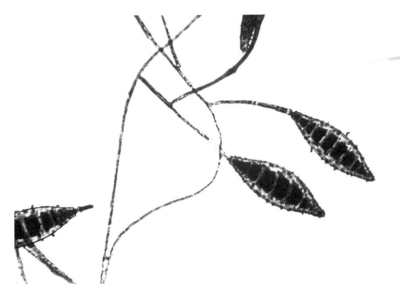

FIGURE 5.6 Microscopic image of *Microsporum canis* macroconidia.

5.4. RESULTS

Fungal culture performed on skin scrapings of this patient grew the mould, *Microsporum canis*, which frequently infects dogs, domestic cats, and ferrets. Unfortunately, the pets are often asymptomatic carriers. After consultation with the pediatrician, the family had all of the pets tested for ringworm, and all three cats were positive for *M. canis*.

5.5. PATHOGENESIS

Our patient has been diagnosed with a dermatophyte infection. Dermatophytes are keratinophilic organisms that grow on nails, hair, and skin. Moulds that cause ringworm produce massive amounts of asexual spores that are carried on desquamated skin scales, and infection occurs by contact with spores shed from animals (zoophilic), humans (anthropophilic), or soil (geophilic). Species of dermatophytes that infect animals (dogs, cats, cattle, horses, goats, poultry) can easily be transmitted to humans. Occupations or hobbies requiring handling of soil, such as gardening or farming, are higher risk for exposure to the spores of these fungi. Public bathing areas, gym showers, and close quarters, such as military camps, are places where infections are commonly acquired.

Direct contact with an infected person or animal is not required for transmission. The fungal spores (vegetative cells with thick walls) can survive in the environment for over a year. These fungal cells adhere to keratinocytes, germinate, and then invade the skin tissue, hair, or nail. Dermatophytes secrete proteinases that aid in penetration of the host cells. Individual susceptibility to dermatophytes renders some people more vulnerable to infection.

Development of delayed-type hypersensitivity correlates with recovery. T-cell activation is critical to resolve the infection, and neutrophils are not commonly seen as part of the inflammatory response. Our patient most likely acquired his infection from his cats, which also tested positive for *M. canis*. He is an immunocompetent host, and with appropriate therapy, his infection cleared.

5.6. TREATMENT AND PREVENTION

Topical antifungal therapy is effective for most skin infections with dermatophytes. Useful topical antifungals include terbinafine, clotrimazole, ketoconazole, and miconazole. Hair and nail infection are best treated with oral drugs, such as terbinafine, itraconazole, and fluconazole. Although griseofulvin has been an acceptable treatment for tinea capitis for many years, it has been replaced by terbinafine or itraconazole which are used to treat nail infections (onychomycosis). Topical therapy for most dermatophyte infections requires many weeks of application, but the newer oral agents may cure the infection in a week. Because the oral therapy is more expensive, microscopic or culture confirmation is often required by health insurance companies before they will reimburse for the treatment.

It is important to determine the organism causing scalp infections because if it is of human origin, it may spread to other close contacts, such as children in a classroom. Zoophilic species don't spread from person to person, but if several family members have the same animal exposure, they may also develop the disease. All the children and adults in this family should be checked for fungal lesions from close contact with their cats.

There is no vaccine to prevent dermatophyte infections. In most cases it is more of an annoyance than an acute medical concern.

5.7. ADDITIONAL POINTS

■ Diagnosis of dermatophyte infections of the hair can be made with the use of a Wood's light, a black light of short ultraviolet wavelength. *Microsporum* spp. fluoresce blue-green when exposed to the light (Fig. 5.7); *Trichophyton* spp. and *Epidermatophyton* spp. will not fluoresce.

■ Tinea versicolor is a fungal infection that affects mainly the skin of young people. Spots and/or rings are light or reddish-brown but always lighter than the surrounding skin. The causative agent is a fat-loving (lipophilic) yeast, called *Malassezia furfur*, which is normal skin flora for humans. The predilection for fat-containing areas of the skin explains why tinea versicolor is common on areas of the body that have many sebaceous (oil) glands such as the chest, back, and shoulders (Fig. 5.8).

■ Outbreaks of tinea corporis have occurred in several athletic teams. In one report, ten members of a high school wrestling team presented with tinea corporis, and the skin lesions matched areas of closest contact with fellow wrestlers. Because there have been so many reports of such tinea spread among members of wrestling teams, this phenomenon is now known as "tinea corporis gladiatorum."

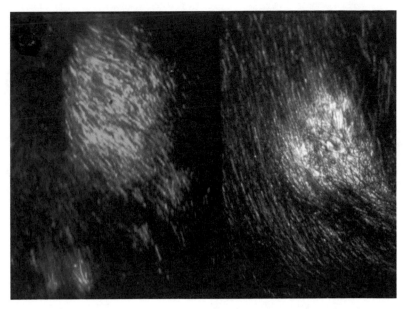

FIGURE 5.7 Wood's light reaction positive (left), negative (right).

■ Cutaneous or dermal larva migrans is the second most common helminth infection in developed countries (pinworm is number 1). It presents as a serpiginous cutaneous eruption confined to the skin of the feet, arms, or buttocks and is caused by the larvae of dog and cat hookworms, which are roundworms (nematodes). The eggs of dog and cat hookworms hatch after being passed in the animal's feces, and humans

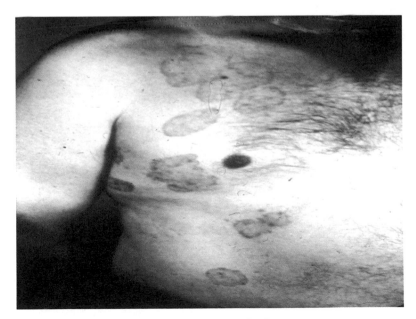

FIGURE 5.8 Tinea versicolor lesions.

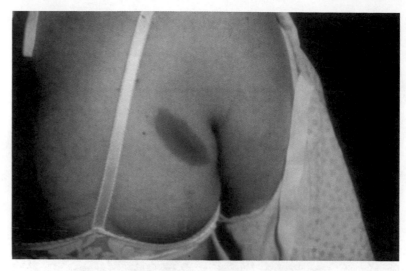

FIGURE 5.9 Erythema migrans rash of Lyme disease.

are infected when these larvae penetrate the skin. The migration of the larvae produces a 2–4-mm wide red, elevated, vesicular track.

- When bacterial and fungal cultures are negative, two noninfectious causes should be considerered: granuloma annulare and nummular eczema. Granuloma annulare is a chronic skin disease consisting of a rash with reddish bumps arranged in a circle or ring. Granuloma annulare most often affects children and young adults and it is slightly more common in girls. Nummular eczema is a stubborn, sometimes itchy rash that forms coin-shaped lesions on the skin. As they age, the lesions may clear in the center, resembling ringworm. The condition tends to be chronic, and the cause is unknown.

- Although Lyme disease is associated with circular skin lesions, the "bulls-eye lesion" of Lyme has a red center that differs from the clear center lesion seen in dermatophyte infections (Fig. 5.9).

SUGGESTED READING

BORGERS, M., H. DEGREEF, AND G. CAUWEN-BERGH, Fungal infections of the skin: Infection process and anti-mycotic therapy, *Curr. Drug Targets* **6**: 849–862 (2005).

HAINER, B. L., Dermatophyte infections, *Am. Fam. Physician* **67**: 101–108 (2003).

WEINSTEIN, A. AND B. BERMAN, Topical treatment of common superficial tinea infections, *Am. Fam. Physician* **65**: 2095–2102 (2002).

Student with a Skin Lesion Following a Trip to India

6.1. PATIENT HISTORY

The patient is a 22 year-old female from southern India who attends a small liberal arts college in Virginia. Two weeks after returning from spring break, she presented to a local emergency department complaining of a painless ulcerative skin lesion with impressive surrounding edema on her left hand. Except for axillary lymphadenopathy on her left side, she was afebrile, had no other constitutional symptoms, and had a benign physical exam. She remarked to physicians that she had originally thought the lesion to be an insect bite, because it started as a raised and very itchy bump before developing into a vesicle and then a painless ulcer, which then formed a black scab. Because she had returned home to India during the break, an infectious disease consult was ordered. On further questioning, she revealed that she had brought several untanned sheep and goat skins from home because she designs and sews coin purses for her friends at school. She has been working with the skins intensely (soaking, stretching, cutting, stitching, and staining) in a studio in the college art department since returning to school.

6.2. DIFFERENTIAL DIAGNOSIS

The differential for infectious diseases with dermatologic findings is enormous, but in some cases, skin lesions are the only visible findings that aid

Medical Microbiology for the New Curriculum: A Case-Based Approach, by Roberta B. Carey, Mindy G. Schuster, and Karin L. McGowan.
Copyright © 2008 John Wiley & Sons, Inc.

the clinician in making a diagnosis. Skin disorders are frequently acquired by travelers and may be due to a wide range of organisms. This patient not only traveled to southern India but also had exposure to untreated animal skins. Both of these risk factors need to be taken into account when considering the differential diagnosis.

Infectious Causes

Bacteria

Aeromonas spp.

Bacillus anthracis

Burkholderia mallei and *B. pseudomallei* (if patient has traveled in SE Asia)

Corynebacterium diphtheriae (if patient is unimmunized)

Erysipelothrix rhusiopathiae

Francisella tularensis

Mycobacterium marinum

Mycobacterium ulcerans

Rickettsia infections

Staphylococcus aureus

Streptococcus pyogenes (necrotizing fasciitis)

Vibrio vulnificus

Yersinia pestis

Viruses

Herpes simplex virus

Orf virus (a viral infection of animals acquired through close contact)

Fungi

Blastomyces dermatitidis

Coccidioides immitis

Cryptococcus neoformans

Histoplasma capsulatum

Paracoccidioides brasiliensis

Sporothrix schenckii

Zygomycetes (*Mucor, Rhizopus,* etc.)

Parasites

Arthropod bites

Dracunculus spp.

Entamoeba histolytica (usually very painful)

Leishmania spp.

Noninfectious Causes

Foreign body

Trauma

Vasculitis

CLINICAL CLUES

[?] Redness, swelling, and pus at a wound site within 48 h following trauma? Think common bacterial causes of infection—staphylococci and streptococci.

[?] Purplish skin infection with bullae formation following contact with brackish water? Think gram-negative rods, such as *Aeromonas* or *Vibrio* (these patients are often systemically ill).

[?] Wound infection following dog or cat bite or scratch? Think *Pasteurella multocida* or *Capnocytophaga canimorsus* (DF-2), a gram-negative rod. Human bites contain a more diverse mix of bacteria and may be worse than an animal bite.

[?] A chronic infection at the site of liposuction? Think rapidly growing mycobacteria, which may not respond to common antimicrobial agents.

[?] Excessive edema for the size of the wound? Painless lesion with black eschar? Think *Bacillus anthracis*.

6.3. LABORATORY TESTS

Because of the enormous amount of edema surrounding the skin lesion on this patient and her exposure to animal skins obtained from southern India, the local department of health was contacted immediately, and the diagnosis of cutaneous anthrax (*B. anthracis*) was strongly suspected. Blood cultures and Gram stain of the skin lesion are high-yield tests in patients with cutaneous anthrax who have not taken antibiotics. A Gram stain is the easiest and fastest way to initially identify suspected cases. *B. anthracis* appears as a large gram-positive spore-forming rod. With cutaneous anthrax, the organism can be isolated from blood, skin lesion, and punch biopsy cultures. If the skin lesion is in the vesicular stage, fluid from intact vesicles should be collected on a sterile swab(s). If the skin lesion appears as a dark black scab (eschar) (Fig. 6.1), then without removing the scab, one should insert a sterile swab moistened with sterile saline underneath the edge, rotate, and collect the lesion material. All specimens suspected of containing bioterrorism agents such as *B. anthracis* must be hand-carried to the laboratory. Pneumatic tube transport systems should never be used. Because Gram stain and culture may not be definitive, multiple (two or three) punch biopsy specimens from the lesion should be taken for histology, culture, and polymerase chain reaction (PCR) testing. State public health laboratories are prepared to perform PCR for *B. anthracis* and other agents of bioterrorism within hours of receiving the

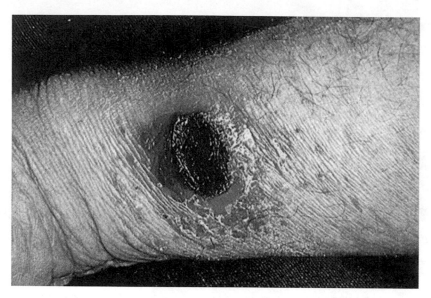

FIGURE 6.1 Eschar lesion.

specimens. Of course, all laboratories should be appropriately notified that a bioterrorism agent is suspected. With suspected bioterrorism organisms, all clinical laboratory specimens must be handled in Biosafety Level 2 facilities. If this is not possible, then all specimens should be transported to the nearest state public health laboratory.

Multiple biopsy specimens and swabs were obtained from the skin ulcer on this patient. Three sets of blood cultures were also obtained, and the patient was admitted and placed in an isolation room. While cutaneous anthrax was strongly suspected in this patient, aerobic and anaerobic bacterial cultures as well as fungal cultures were requested on all specimens to allow for additional pathogens. Skin ulcer and biopsy specimens were also transported to the state public health laboratory for PCR testing.

6.4. RESULTS

Gram stains performed on the cutaneous lesion specimens were positive for large gram-positive rods. Skin swabs and biopsy specimens were both positive for *B. anthracis* by PCR. All three blood cultures as well as bacterial wound cultures grew gram-positive rods within 24 h (Fig. 6.2). Several critical characteristics aid in the presumptive laboratory identification of *B. anthracis*. The organism is characterized by being a gram-positive, spore-forming rod (Fig. 6.3), by the absence of hemolysis on sheep blood agar (Fig. 6.4), and by lack of motility and lack of growth on phenylethyl alcohol (PEA) medium. Suspected isolates are then confirmed by PCR at state public health laboratories.

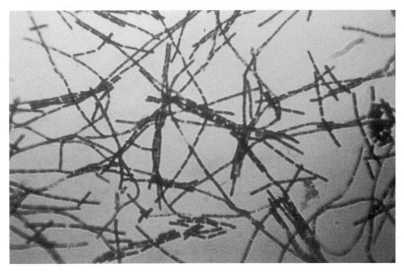

FIGURE 6.2 Gram stain showing chaining gram-positive rods.

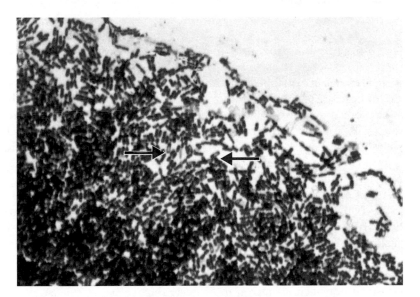

FIGURE 6.3 Gram stain showing gram-positive rods with spores.

6.5. PATHOGENESIS

Persons with occupational exposure to animal hides, hair, or the wool of infected animals may contract the cutaneous or respiratory form of anthrax. Skin infections may begin as a bump at the site of an abrasion or cut, where the spores enter the tissue. A fluid-filled vesicle with numerous organisms matures into a painless ulcer with a black center (eschar) over a short period of time (2–3 days). The cutaneous infection may become systemic, and death may result from acute respiratory distress. A primary respiratory infection (inhalation anthrax) presents with signs and symptoms similar to

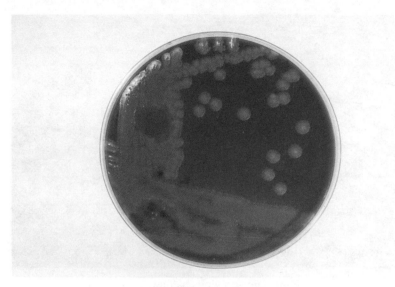

FIGURE 6.4 Nonhemolytic colonies of *Bacillus anthracis* on blood agar.

those of influenza, but progresses to respiratory distress and is often fatal. Mortality approaches 100% in patients with the later stages of the disease. Physical findings are nonspecific, although the chest x-ray in patients with respiratory anthrax is pathognomonic—a widened mediastinum with or without pleural effusions. Humans who ingest contaminated meat may acquire gastrointestinal anthrax, characterized by nausea, vomiting, fever with abdominal pain, and bloody diarrhea, which are nonspecific symptoms for gastrointestinal infection due to many foodborne pathogens.

All virulent strains of *B. anthracis* have a capsule that allows the organism to resist phagocytosis. The genes that control expression of the capsule are located on a plasmid. A second plasmid contains the genes for exotoxin production. Three key components must be present for the total expression of virulence: (1) protective antigen (PA), which binds to the host cell; (2) edema factor (EF, adenyl cyclase), which causes fluid accumulation; and (3) lethal factor (LF), a zinc metalloprotease that stimulates macrophages to release tumor necrosis factor and interleukin 1. Excess release of these immune response factors leads to cell death:

PA + EF → edema toxin

PA + LF → lethal toxin

Capsule + edema toxin + lethal toxin → → *a virulent organism*

After a person is exposed to anthrax through skin, respiratory, or gastrointestinal contact, the spores are engulfed by macrophages, where they become vegetative bacilli that multiply within the macrophage until the macrophage bursts, releasing the bacteria into the bloodstream. The bacteria release a PA toxin that binds to host cell receptors. A cluster of seven of these PA molecules forms a hollow sphere where another toxin (EF or LF) may bind in the core. The entire sphere is surrounded by the cell membrane and taken into the cell cytoplasm, where the toxins are released and the cell is destroyed.

The combination of having several virulence factors and the ability to survive harsh environmental conditions in spore form makes *B. anthracis* a very effective pathogen. These characteristics also enable *B. anthracis* to be a very effective bioweapon for use in bioterrorism (BT) attacks. Because of the heightened awareness of anthrax as a BT agent, any infection with this organism is considered to have a BT origin until proven otherwise. However, natural infections do occur, as in the case of our patient, who handled infected hides from animals contaminated with the organism. Human-to-human transmission of anthrax is extremely unlikely, and even animal-to-animal transmission within a species is unusual.

6.6. TREATMENT AND PREVENTION

Our patient was treated with a course of ciprofloxacin, a fluoroquinolone with good tissue penetration. Treatment options for anthrax infections include penicillin, doxycycline, or ciprofloxacin, all of which can be administered orally. *B. anthracis* is resistant to sulfonamides and extended-spectrum cephalosporins. Ciprofloxacin has been given as empiric therapy in case of a BT event since experiments have shown that the organism could be genetically engineered to be resistant to penicillin and doxycycline. Ciprofloxacin is also the antimicrobial of choice for post-exposure prophylaxis. The administration of antibiotics prevents the development of protective antibodies, and the risk for recurrent infection remains for ≤60 days because of the delayed germination of the bacterial spores. This prophyaxis regimen may be shortened to 30–45 days when coupled with concomitant anthrax vaccine.

Vaccination with an avirulent, nonencapsulated, live strain of *B. anthracis* is used to control disease in herbivorous livestock (cattle, sheep, goats, antelope), which may ingest spores that persist in the soil for decades. However, underdeveloped countries cannot afford to vaccinate their livestock, so anthrax is endemic in their animal populations. Humans who work with animals or animal products, those in the military, and laboratorians who work with virulent strains of *B. anthracis* should be vaccinated with a cell-free vaccine. Human vaccine and antibiotics are stockpiled in the event of a bioterrorist attack. Because person-to-person transmission has not occurred, no treatment or immunization of household contacts is required unless they were exposed to the same source of infection.

6.7. ADDITIONAL POINTS

■ Whenever potential agents of bioterrorism (*Bacillus anthracis, Burkholderia mallei, Burkholderia pseudomallei, Francisella tularensis, Yersinia pestis*) are suspected or presumptively identified by a laboratory, regional public health officials should be notified immediately.

- The most common diagnoses of skin lesions following travel are arthropod-reactive dermatitis, cutaneous larva migrans, cutaneous leishmaniasis, fly maggot infestation (myiasis), burrowing fleas (tungiasis), and hives (urticaria).

- When *B. anthracis, Y. pestis, F. tularensis,* or *Brucella* species are recovered from a patient, it is important to establish a history of exposure to animals that carry these microorganisms to separate a naturally occurring infection from a possible bioterrorism event.

SUGGESTED READING

CDC, CDC anthrax investigation updates and new information, *MMWR* **50**:1–4 (2001).

CDC, Inhalation anthrax associated with dried animal hides—Pennsylvania and New York City, *MMWR* **55**:280–282 (2006).

DAYA, M. AND Y. NAKAMURA, Pulmonary disease from biological agents: Anthrax, plague, Q fever, and tularemia, *Crit. Care Clin.* **21**: 747–763 (2005).

HOLTY, J. E., D. M. BRAVATA, H. LIU, R. A. OLSHEN, K. M. MCDONALD, AND D. K. OWENS, Systematic review: A century of inhalational anthrax cases from 1900 to 2005, *Ann. Intern. Med.* **144**:270–280 (2006).

JAMA Consensus Statement, Anthrax as a biological weapon: Medical and public health management, *JAMA* **281**:1735–1745 (1999).

Man with a Surgical Wound after a Prosthetic Hip Placement

7.1. PATIENT HISTORY

A 72 year-old man with a history of rheumatoid arthritis underwent placement of a prosthetic left total hip two weeks ago. The wound initially started healing, but over the past 3–4 days, he noted increasing pain in the joint with redness and swelling. Yesterday, he noted a small blister over the middle of the incision, and today that area has opened up and begun to drain purulent material. He denies any fever or chills. On physical examination, he is well-appearing, but has difficulty bearing weight on his left leg because of pain. His temperature is 38°C (100.4°F), heart rate 86 beats/min , blood pressure 180/78 mm Hg, and respiratory rate 18 breaths/min . There are no oral or skin lesions. His chest is clear. Cardiac exam is without murmurs, rubs, or gallops. The remainder of the exam is unremarkable, except for his left leg. There is severe pain on rotation of his hip. The incision is warm, erythematous, hard (indurated), and tender. There is a small area where the skin has split open (dehiscence) where purulent material can be expressed. Laboratory studies reveal a white blood cell count of $11.8/mm^3$, and normal electrolytes. The erythrocyte sedimentation rate (ESR) is 86 mm/h. Plain radiographs of the left hip are unremarkable. A joint aspirate yielded 20 mL of thick cloudy fluid.

Medical Microbiology for the New Curriculum: A Case-Based Approach, by Roberta B. Carey, Mindy G. Schuster, and Karin L. McGowan.

7.2. DIFFERENTIAL DIAGNOSIS

Wound infections contribute significantly to morbidity and mortality following surgery. Post-operative wound infections are frequently polymicrobial in nature, and the risk of acquiring a postoperative wound infection increases with prolonged operating time, the nature of the surgery (clean vs. dirty), increased number of blood transfusions, and the length of hospital stay. Organisms causing wound infections stem from three main sources: the environment (hospital operating room and staff), the surrounding skin (patient's endogenous flora), and, if appropriate, the closest endogenous mucous membrane.

Infectious Causes

Organisms responsible for postoperative wound infections following prosthetic joint replacement include those listed below.

Bacteria

Anaerobes—including *Bacteroides* spp., *Clostridium* spp., and anaerobic cocci

Enterococcus spp.

Gram-negative rods—including *Enterobacteriaceae*, *Pseudomonas* spp., and *Stenotrophomonas maltophilia*

Staphylococcus aureus

Staphylococcus spp.—coagulase-negative

Streptococcus spp.—including β-hemolytic streptococci, *S. pneumoniae*, *S. milleri*, and other viridans streptococci

Fungi

Candida albicans and other *Candida* species

Parasites

Parasites are not a cause of postoperative wound infections.

Viruses

Viruses are not a cause of postoperative wound infections.

CLINICAL CLUES

? Blister over incision? Think staphylococci or streptococci.

? Is the site warm, erythematous, swollen, or tender, and is a discharge present? Staphylococcal infection is very likely.

? Is there an odor present? Sweet, fruity smell implies *Pseudomonas*; putrid odor implies anaerobes.

? On palpation of the site, is crepitance (crackling sound) present? This is from gas production and implicates anaerobes or gram-negative rods.

7.3. LABORATORY TESTS

Because of the wide variety of bacteria involved in wound infections, both routine bacterial cultures and anaerobic cultures should be requested in addition to a Gram stain of the purulent material. In patients such as this one where a major joint is affected, joint fluid must also be submitted for routine and anaerobic culture, cell count, and differential. In a febrile patient suspected of having a wound infection, blood cultures should be performed because wound infections frequently result in bacterial invasion of the bloodstream (bacteremia). Areas to be tested for wound cultures should be cleaned with 70% alcohol before sampling by aspiration or before using swabs moistened with a transport medium to collect material. Wound fluid, aspirates of purulent material, as well as tissue specimens must be delivered promptly to the laboratory (<2 h at room temperature), particularly if anaerobic bacteria are suspected. Special pre-reduced transport media, as well as anaerobic transport vials for swabs, are available to maintain the viability of aerobic and anaerobic bacteria during transport. A swab is not optimal for anaerobic culture; aspirates are preferred. Tissue specimens should be submitted in a sterile container and kept moist during transport to prevent drying. Routine analysis of wound specimens normally involves the use of selective and nonselective culture media that support the growth of aerobic and facultative bacteria, as well as yeasts. Since many of the organisms involved in wound pathology take longer than 48 h to grow, particularly anaerobes, it is not unusual for wound cultures to take 4–5 days to be completed. Performing a Gram stain on abscess, fluid, or tissue material is critical since the presence of many polymorphonuclear neutrophils (PMNs) helps to support the diagnosis of a wound infection. In addition, because culture results are not immediately available, clinical clues as well as Gram stain findings may help in the choice of antibiotics used in treatment.

7.4. RESULTS

The joint fluid cell count and differential revealed that the fluid contained 100,000 WBC/mm^3, 80% PMNs, and 20% lymphocytes. Gram stain of the purulent joint fluid revealed many WBC and gram-positive cocci in clusters (Fig. 7.1). Bacterial colonies present on 5% sheep blood agar after 24 h incubation appeared smooth, raised, cream-yellow, and glistening with a zone of β-hemolysis suggestive of a staphylococcus (Fig. 7.2). Gram stain of the colony showed gram-positive cocci in grape-like clusters, which is suggestive of staphylococci. On Gram stain, streptococci and enterococci appear as gram-positive cocci in chains (Fig. 7.3). No anaerobes were isolated.

In the identification of gram-positive cocci, the first biochemical test performed is usually the catalase test, which uses 3% hydrogen peroxide (H$_2$O$_2$). Staphylococci are catalase-positive and exhibit bubbling when mixed with H$_2$O$_2$ (Fig. 7.4). Streptococci and enterococci are catalase-negative and do not produce bubbles. The coagulase test is the primary test used to distinguish coagulase-positive *Staphylococcus aureus* from the coagulase-negative staphylococci (CoNS). *S. aureus* produce two types of

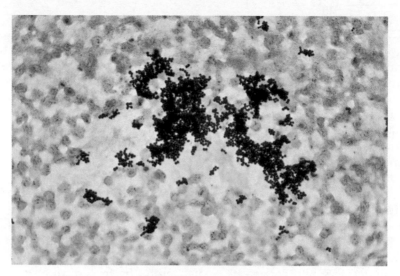

FIGURE 7.1 Gram stain of gram-positive cocci in clusters.

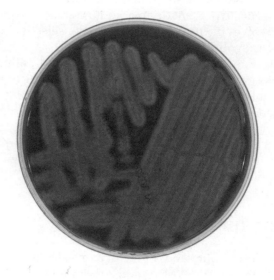

FIGURE 7.2 β-Hemolytic colonies on blood agar plate.

coagulase: bound coagulase, which is also called "clumping factor," which is bound to the bacterial cell wall and directly reacts with fibrinogen; and free coagulase, which clots plasma when inoculated and incubated with *S. aureus* colonies in the tube coagulase test (Fig. 7.5). A rapid slide latex agglutination test that detects both bound coagulase and/or protein A on the surface of staphylococci is also available, and *S. aureus* possesses both factors (Fig. 7.6). This patient's bacterial isolate was both catalase- and coagulase-positive and was identified as *S. aureus*.

Antibiotic susceptibility test results showed this patient's *S. aureus* isolate to be resistant to ampicillin/sulbactam, cefazolin, cefotaxime, cefuroxime, ciprofloxacin, clindamycin, erythromycin, imipenem, oxacillin,

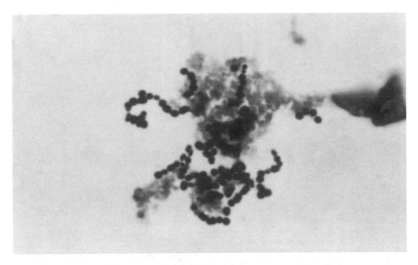

FIGURE 7.3 Gram stain of gram-positive cocci in chains.

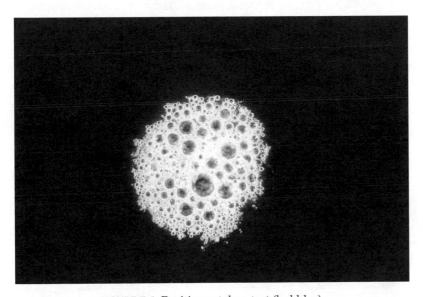

FIGURE 7.4 Positive catalase test (bubbles).

and penicillin. The isolate was susceptible to vancomycin, trimethoprim–sulfamethoxazole, linezolid, and quinupristin/dalfopristin. A broth microtiter dilution test was performed in the laboratory to detect antimicrobial susceptibility (Fig. 7.7). Serial twofold dilutions of each antimicrobial agent are inoculated with a standardized inoculum of the bacteria and grown overnight in Mueller–Hinton broth. The minimum inhibitory concentration (MIC) is read as the lowest concentration of the antibiotic that inhibits the growth of the bacteria. This is the first well where you see no turbidity or growth of the bacteria. The MICs (μg/mL) are then interpreted for each antimicrobial agent as susceptible, intermediate, or resistant in accordance with standardized guidelines. Since this isolate tested resistant

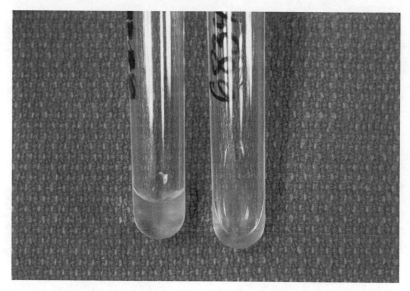

FIGURE 7.5 Positive (left) and negative (right) tube coagulase test.

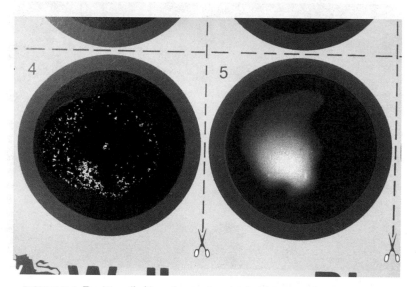

FIGURE 7.6 Positive (left) and negative (right) latex agglutination test.

to one penicillinase-resistant penicillin (oxacillin), it is by definition resistant to all other penicillinase-resistant penicillins. These isolates are called methicillin-resistant *S. aureus* (MRSA).

7.5. PATHOGENESIS

S. aureus is one of the most commonly recognized pathogens causing human and animal disease, but it may be present on or in the body without causing illness. Approximately 25% of the population will harbor *S. aureus* in their noses without any symptoms or infection. However, nasal

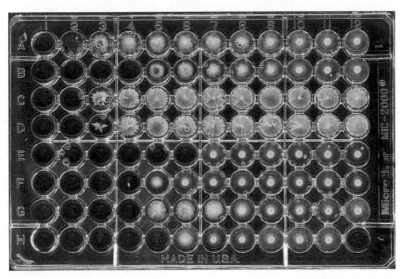

FIGURE 7.7 Antibiotic susceptibility test by broth microdilution method.

carriage can increase a person's risk for staphylococcal infection. *S. aureus* can spread person to person, due to close contact to an infected person, or through indirect contact by touching objects, such as towels or sports equipment that has come in contact with the skin of a person infected with *S. aureus*. Infections occur when the skin or mucosal barriers are compromised, allowing access of the staphylococci to adjoining tissues or the bloodstream. The risk of infection is increased by the presence of a foreign body, such as a prosthetic device or a catheter, since phagocytic function is diminished at those sites.

The staphylococcal components and products that make *S. aureus* an effective pathogen are listed in Table 7.1.

Our patient had a joint infection that was the result of contiguous spread from a wound infection, or more likely, contamination at the time of joint placement. *S. aureus* causes infection of the heart valves (endocarditis), infection of the bones (osteomyelitis), and toxic shock syndrome where the function of all organs (lungs, kidney, heart) is shut down because of the activity of toxic shock syndrome toxin (TSST-1). TSST-1 causes an expansion of the T cells, resulting in a massive release of cytokines by macrophages and T cells. The incidence of staphylococcal toxic shock syndrome increased in 1985 with the introduction of superabsorbent tampons. Patients presented with high fever, rash, hypotension, and multiorgan system failure. Since the withdrawal of these tampons from the market, toxic shock syndrome is associated more often with localized skin infections, surgery, or insect bites.

7.6. TREATMENT AND PREVENTION

Only 5% of the *S. aureus* strains in the United States remain susceptible to penicillin since most *S. aureus* produce a β-lactamase that destroys the activity of penicillin and its derivatives, such as ampicillin, amoxicillin,

TABLE 7.1.	Virulence Factors of *S. aureus* and Their Mechanism of Action
Virulence Factor	Action Mechanism
Cell wall peptidoglycan	Endotoxin-like activity Stimulates release of cytokines Activates complement Aggregates platelets
Capsular polysaccharide	Antiphagocytic
Surface proteins	Adhesins to colonize host tissue
Protein A	Antiphagocytic
Pyrogenic–toxin superantigens	Cause T-cell proliferation Cytokine release Causes toxic shock syndrome
Enterotoxin	Food poisoning
Exfoliative toxins	Cause skin erythema and separation
Panton–Valentine leukocidin	Causes severe cutaneous infections
Protease, lipase, hyaluronidase	Facilitates spread of infection to adjoining tissues

ticarcillin, and piperacillin. Therefore, this very effective class of antimicrobials has lost its place in routine treatment of staphylococcal infections. If the patient's organisms are tested in vitro and demonstrate susceptibility to oxacillin, then one of the semisynthetic penicillins (oxacillin, nafcillin, dicloxacillin) can be used. Alternative antibiotics, ampicillin/sulbactam, and first-generation cephalosporins, are effective if the *S. aureus* is oxacillin-susceptible; however, these drugs will be reported as resistant if laboratory tests indicate that the isolate is resistant to oxacillin (MRSA).

Staphylococcal resistance to methicillin/oxacillin occurs when organisms have an altered penicillin-binding protein, PBP2a, which is encoded by the *mecA* gene. The alteration of the penicillin-binding protein does not allow the antibiotic to bind well to the bacterial cell, leading to resistance to all β-lactam antimicrobial agents. This resistance determinant is carried on a mobile genetic element called the staphylococcal cassette chromosome *mec* (SCC*mec*). SCC*mec* IV is associated with community-acquired infections, while SCC*mec* I and II are most often associated with hospital-acquired staphylococcal infections.

Accurate laboratory detection of methicillin/oxacillin resistance can be difficult since the population of staphylococci consists of both susceptible and resistant subpopulations that coexist in the culture. Intravenous vancomycin is the treatment of choice for serious infections caused by MRSA. Newer antimicrobials, quinopristin/dalfopristin, and linezolid are also active against strains of MRSA. More worrisome is the increase of vancomycin intermediate and vancomycin-resistant *S. aureus* (VISA, VRSA) that have arisen in the last few years. High-level vancomycin resistance has been acquired by the insertion of the *vanA* gene from enterococci into *S. aureus*. Vancomycin intermediate strains are a result of a change in the cell wall composition, which prevents the binding of the antibiotic to the cell wall.

MRSA are seen most commonly as a hospital-acquired pathogen. In many hospitals, up to 50% of *S. aureus* are MRSA. Because of the limited numbers of antimicrobials available to treat MRSA, our patient will be put on "contact precautions" to minimize the transmission of this resistant microorganism to other patients. These infection control guidelines include a private room or cohorting our patient with other patients with MRSA. Healthcare personnel must wear a gown and clean, nonsterile gloves when entering the room and caring for the patient. The gown and gloves must be removed when the healthcare worker exits the room, and hands must be washed with an antimicrobial agent or a waterless antiseptic. There should be limited movement of the patient to other areas of the hospital, and noncritical equipment should be dedicated to the patient and not shared with others. Those at higher risk for acquiring MRSA include patients with prolonged hospital stay, those receiving broad-spectrum antibiotics, those hospitalized in intensive care units, those with recent surgery, or patients carrying MRSA in their noses.

Community-associated MRSA is found in people with no recent contact to hospitals or long-term care centers. Severe skin infections have been seen in those incarcerated in prisons and jails; males who play close contact sports, such as football, wrestling or fencing; children in daycare; drug users; and men who have sex with men. Physicians in the community must be aware that MRSA may be found in these populations and treat skin infections accordingly with appropriate antimicrobials. There is no vaccine to protect those at risk from acquiring MRSA.

7.7. ADDITIONAL POINTS

- The top six pathogens isolated from postsurgical wounds from all types of surgery are *S. aureus*, CoNS, *Enterococcus* spp., *Escherichia coli*, *Pseudomonas aeruginosa*, and *Enterobacter* spp.

- CoNS are normal flora on human skin and mucous membranes. They can also be significant opportunistic pathogens because of their ability to adhere to and grow on plastic and polymer surfaces, due to their production of a mucoid slime like material in vivo. CoNS have emerged as primary pathogens capable of causing infections of indwelling devices (catheters, shunts, prosthetics, etc.), postsurgical endophthalmitis, endocarditis, urinary tract infections, and bacteremia in immunosuppressed hosts. While *Staphylococcus epidermidis* is the species causing over 80% of CoNS infections, almost all species have been reported to cause infection in humans.

- Mycobacteria other than *M. tuberculosis* (MOTT) should be considered in the differential when late-onset postsurgical infections are seen, particularly following plastic surgery. These infections are not as acute because this group of bacteria is more indolent and slow-growing.

SUGGESTED READING

BARBERAN, J., Management of infections of osteoarticular prosthesis, *Clin. Microbiol. Infect.* **12**(Suppl. 3):93–101 (2006).

CUNHA, B. A., Methicillin-resistant *Staphylococcus aureus*: Clinical manifestations and antimicrobial therapy, *Clin. Microbiol. Infect.* **11**(Suppl. 4):33–42 (2005).

GARNER, J. S., Hospital Infection Control Practice Advisory Committee (HICPAC) Guidelines for isolation precautions in hospitals, *Infect. Control Hosp. Epi.* **17**:53–80 (1996).

www.cdc.gov/ncidod/hip/isolat.

GORDON, S. M., Antibiotic prophylaxis against postoperative wound infections, *Clev. Clin. J. Med.* **73**(Suppl. 1):S42–S45 (2006).

www.cdc.gov/ncidod/hip/ARESIST/mrsafaq. htm.

ZIMMERLI, W., A. TRAMPUZ, AND P. E. OCHSNER, Prosthetic-joint infections, *N. Engl. J. Med.* **351**:1645–1654 (2004).

Boy with Fever and Right Leg Pain Following a Canoe Accident

8.1. PATIENT HISTORY

This case concerns a previously healthy 13 year-old male complaining of pain and stiffness in his right knee and leg. Three weeks prior to presentation he was involved in a canoeing accident at a boy scout camp resulting in an open wound on his right (R) leg. When he returned home 10 days later, the surface skin wound had healed but he complained of R knee and leg pain with nausea and vomiting. When examined by his pediatrician, he was febrile and had a raised pulse of 120 beats/min. Petechiae were noted on his R leg, and flexing the R knee caused severe pain. He was taken to the local hospital emergency department, where on physical exam he had a fever of 39°C (102.2°F), blood pressure of 93/58 mm Hg, and heart rate of 98 beats/min. No areas of palpable lymphadenopathy were found. He appeared alert, responsive, well nourished, and nontoxic. Edema was noted in his right tibia, the right knee was warm to the touch, but he had full range of motion and walked without difficulty. Immunizations were up-to-date, and he had never been hospitalized previously. There was no travel history and no pet exposure. Initial laboratory results included a WBC count of 14,600/mm^3 with 65% segmented neutrophils, 4% band forms, and 31% lymphocytes. Hemoglobin was 12 g/dL, hematocrit was 35%, and the platelet count was 280,000/mm^3. The erythrocyte sedimentation rate (ESR) was 76 mm/h, and the C-reactive protein (CRP) 20 mg/L. Cystic irregularities were noted on x-ray, and a bone scan showed increased uptake in the R tibia. An MRI was read as osteomyelitis with questionable abscess. Blood cultures were taken, and he was admitted for further evaluation.

8.2. DIFFERENTIAL DIAGNOSIS

Osteomyelitis (OM) is an acute or chronic bone and bone marrow infection caused by aerobic and anaerobic bacteria, mycobacteria, and fungi. The organism that causes OM is often causing an infection in another part of the body and spreads to the bone via the bloodstream. OM occurs at sites of bone affected by trauma or surgery, in vertebrae, and in bones of the feet of diabetes patients. In children, OM usually affects growing bones with a rich blood supply and is most commonly seen at the wider part of the shaft of a long bone (metaphysis) such as the tibia or femur. In adults, the vertebrae and the pelvis are most commonly affected. There are three routes of acquiring OM: hematogenous, contiguous from an adjacent infection site, and direct inoculation of organisms into bone or nearby tissue by trauma, surgery, IV drug use, or open bone fractures. The most common form, acute hematogenous OM, occurs primarily in young children and is most frequently caused by gram-positive organisms. In contrast, direct inoculation and contiguous OM are more common in adults and adolescents. Chronic OM usually results when the diagnosis and treatment of acute OM has been delayed or the OM has not been treated successfully. Chronic infection can persist intermittently for years and is often polymicrobial and very difficult to eradicate. *Staphylococcus epidermidis, S. aureus, Escherichia coli, Serratia marcescens, Pseudomonas aeruginosa,* fungi, and mycobacteria are commonly isolated in patients with chronic OM.

Infectious Causes

Bacteria

The bacterial pathogens causing acute OM vary on the basis of the patient's age and the mechanism of infection. In addition there are a number of specific risk factors that predispose a patient to OM with a specific organism. The age groups are listed below.

Neonates (<6 weeks)

Candida spp.

Enterobacteriaceae

Staphylococcus aureus

Streptococcus agalactiae (group B strep)

Streptococcus spp.

Infants (<1 year)

Haemophilus influenzae

Kingella kingae

Staphylococcus aureus

Streptococcus pneumoniae

Streptococcus pyogenes (group A strep)

Children (1–16 years)

Haemophilus influenzae

Pseudomonas aeruginosa

Salmonella spp.

Staphylococcus aureus

Streptococcus pyogenes (group A strep)

Streptococcus agalactiae (group B strep)

Adults (>16 years)

Escherichia coli

Pseudomonas aeruginosa

Serratia marcescens

Staphylococcus aureus

Staphylococcus spp. (coagulase-negative)

Viruses

Viruses are not a cause of osteomyelitis.

Fungi

Aspergillus spp.

Blastomyces dermatitidis

Candida spp.

Coccidioides spp.

Cryptococcus neoformans

Histoplasma capsulatum

Sporothrix schenckii

Parasites

Parasites are not a cause of osteomyelitis.

Noninfectious Causes

Bone infarction

Cellulitis

Skeletal cancer

Thrombophlebitis

Risk factors for OM are listed in Table 8.1.

TABLE 8.1. **Specific Risk Factors Associated with Organisms Causing Osteomyelitis**

Risk Factor	Organisms
Foreign-body-associated infection	Coagulase-negative staphylococci *Propionibacterium* sp.
Hemodialysis IV drug use	*Staphylococcus epidermidis* *Staphylococcus aureus* Gram-negative organisms *Candida* spp.
Nosocomial infections	*Enterobacteriaceae* *Pseudomonas aeruginosa*
Sickle cell disease	*Salmonella* species *Streptococcus pneumoniae*
Human bites, fist injuries due to contact with another person's mouth, diabetic foot ulcers, decubitus ulcers	Streptococci *Eikenella corrodens* anaerobic bacteria
Animal bites	*Pasteurella multocida*
Trauma	*Staphylococcus aureus* *Enterobacteriaceae* *Pseudomonas aeruginosa*
Foot puncture wound, wound associated with exposure to fresh water	*Pseudomonas aeruginosa* and other *Pseudomonas* spp. *Aeromonas* spp.
Immunocompromised patients	*Aspergillus* spp. *Mycobacterium avium-intracellulare* *Candida* spp.
Human immunodeficiency virus infection	*Bartonella henselae*
Populations in which tuberculosis is prevalent	*Mycobacterium tuberculosis*
Populations with close contact with ruminant animals (sheep, cattle, goats, swine) or turkeys and other birds	*Brucella* species *Coxiella burnetii* (Q fever)
Populations in which these pathogens are endemic; with these organisms, OM is associated with disseminated disease	*Blastomyces dermatitidis* *Coccidioides immitis* *Histoplasma capsulatum* *Sporothrix schenckii* *Cryptococcus neoformans* *Aspergillus* spp.

CLINICAL CLUES

[?] Patient refuses to bear weight on an extremity? Think osteomyelitis.

[?] Unilateral extremity pain in a previously healthy active individual? Think osteomyelitis.

[?] Recent trauma or puncture wound? Think osteomyelitis.

[?] Chronic draining ulcer over bone? Think chronic osteomyelitis with sinus tract.

8.3. LABORATORY TESTS

The diagnosis of OM is based primarily on clinical findings, the initial history, physical examination, and radiologic and laboratory tests. Histopathologic examination, Gram stain, and aerobic and anaerobic microbiology cultures are critical to the diagnosis of OM and necessary to direct antibiotic treatment. To diagnose a bone infection and identify the organisms causing it, blood cultures ($\times 3$), pus from abscesses (if present), joint fluid, or the bone itself (bone biopsy) are useful specimens to obtain. While blood cultures are positive only in approximately 50% of patients with acute OM, blood cultures should always be taken. If positive, they can eliminate the need to take more invasive specimens, such as a bone biopsy. Sinus drainage material is considered unreliable for diagnosing OM and should not be submitted for culture. If joint fluid is present, the fluid should be aspirated and submitted for cell count with differential, protein, glucose, Gram stain, and culture.

An increased WBC count with a left shift, as well as elevations in the ESR (erythrocyte sedimentation rate) and CRP (C-reactive protein), are frequent findings in acute OM and should be ordered when evaluating a patient.

Blood cultures ($\times 3$) were obtained from this patient, but because of his initial radiologic findings, he was immediately scheduled for a bone biopsy. Bone aspirate material was obtained in the operating room and submitted to the laboratory for Gram stain, plus aerobic and anaerobic bacterial cultures. Specimens must be delivered promptly to the laboratory (<2 h at room temperature), particularly if anaerobic bacteria are suspected. Special prereduced transport media as well as anaerobic transport vials for swabs are available to maintain the viability of aerobic and anaerobic bacteria during transport. A swab is not optimal for anaerobic cultures; aspirates or tissues are preferred. Not only are specimens as critical as bone biopsies or aspirates plated on aerobic and anaerobic agar plates; portions of the specimen are also placed in broth media. Tubes of liquid media such as thioglycollate, eugonic, or brain heart infusion broth encourage the growth of fastidious organisms and support the growth of rare numbers of organisms. Growth in broth media is indicated by the medium changing from clear to cloudy (turbid) (Fig. 8.1). Laboratorians subculture the turbid broth onto a battery of solid agar plates to recover the isolate(s). While this process may require a longer turnaround time, it makes a maximum effort to recover the causative organism.

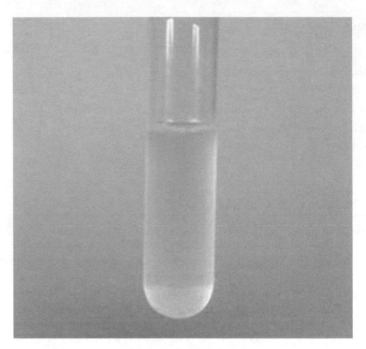

FIGURE 8.1 Turbid broth culture.

8.4. RESULTS

Gram stain of the bone aspirate material revealed WBCs and slender, straight gram-negative rods. After overnight incubation at 35°C, bacterial growth was observed on the aerobic 5% sheep blood agar plate as well as the chocolate agar and MacConkey agar. On the 5% sheep blood agar, the organism was noted to be β-hemolytic (Fig. 8.2). On MacConkey agar the colony was a non-lactose-fermenting gram-negative rod (Fig. 8.3). Further testing showed the gram-negative rod to be oxidase-positive. The oxidase test is used to determine the presence of bacterial cytochrome oxidase using the oxidation of a tetramethyl-p-phenylenediamine dihydrochloride substrate. A positive test shows the development of a dark purple color (oxidase present), and a negative test shows no color development (Fig. 8.4). The isolate was identified as *Pseudomonas aeruginosa* on the basis of its Gram stain morphology, inability to ferment lactose, a positive oxidase reaction, a grape-like fruity odor, and its ability to grow at 42°C. It is the most commonly isolated oxidase-positive gram-negative rod causing human infections.

   P. aeruginosa is an aerobic gram-negative rod, belonging to the family *Pseudomonadaceae*. In comparison to enteric gram-negative rods, which are plump and short, *P. aeruginosa* morphologically appears as a long, slender, straight gram-negative rod (Fig. 8.5). *P. aeruginosa* grows well at 35–37°C on most laboratory media such as 5% sheep blood agar, chocolate agar, or MacConkey agar.

   P. aeruginosa produces two types of soluble pigments, a green fluorescent pigment (fluorescein) and a blue pigment (pyocyanin), which

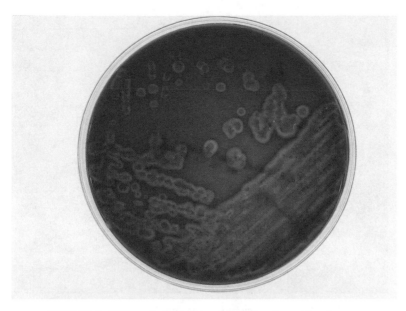

FIGURE 8.2 β-Hemolytic gram-negative rods on blood agar.

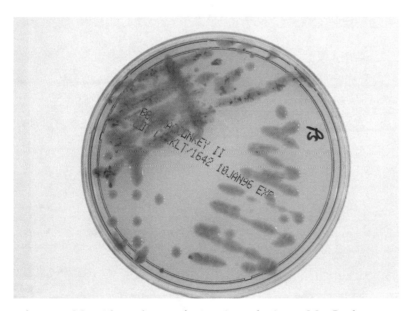

FIGURE 8.3 Mucoid non-lactose fermenting colonies on MacConkey agar

diffuse into media (Fig. 8.6). Fluorescence under ultraviolet light is also helpful in the early identification of *P. aeruginosa* colonies. "Blue pus" is a characteristic of suppurative infections caused by pyocyanin producing *P. aeruginosa* that can actually result in wound dressings turning a blue-green color. Some strains can also produce a red or brown diffusible pigment. *P. aeruginosa* isolates from clinical specimens produce flat or smooth colony types that are β-hemolytic and reveal a metallic sheen on 5% sheep blood agar plates (Fig. 8.7). Strains isolated from patients with cystic

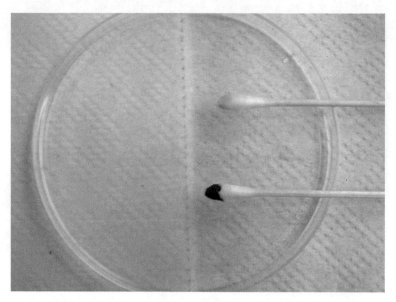

FIGURE 8.4 Oxidase reaction negative (top) positive (bottom).

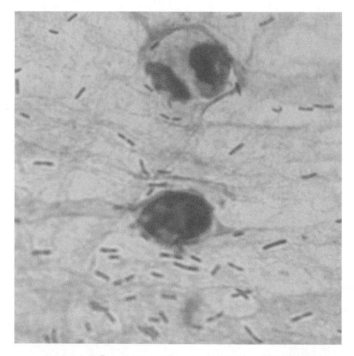

FIGURE 8.5 Gram strain showing gram-negative rods.

fibrosis are extremely mucoid and may not exhibit the characteristic pigment. *P. aeruginosa* is a common inhabitant of water, soil, and plants. The bacterium is ubiquitous in soil and water, and on any surface that has had contact with soil or water. It is rarely isolated from the throats and stools of nonhospitalized patients (2%). Once hospitalized, the gastrointestinal carriage rates rise to 20%.

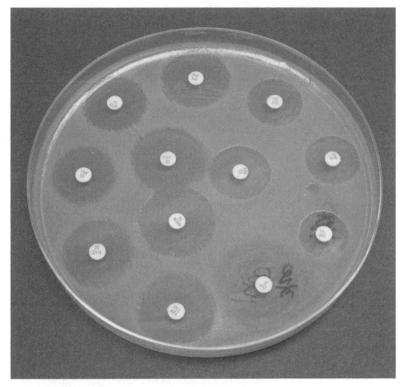

FIGURE 8.6 Pyocyanin (green pigment) of *Pseudomonas aeruginosa*.

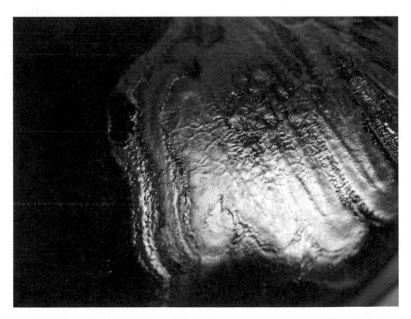

FIGURE 8.7 Metallic sheen of *Pseudomonas aeruginosa* on blood agar.

Antibiotic susceptibility test results showed our patient's *P. aeruginosa* isolate to be susceptible to amikacin, ciprofloxacin, gentamicin, imipenem, piperacillin, ticarcillin, ticarcillin–clavulanic acid, and tobramycin and resistant to aztreonam, cefotaxime, ceftazidime, and chloramphenicol. Anaerobic culture media revealed that no anaerobes were present.

8.5. PATHOGENESIS

Osteomyelitis is characterized by inflammation of bone leading to bone necrosis and formation of dead pieces of bone (sequestrum). When the infection spreads from localized sites to the bone, this frequently results in a polymicrobic infection, while seeding from the blood usually involves a single type of microorganism. For example, diabetics with compromised circulation to their extremities may have chronic soft tissue infections of their feet, which lead to a mixed bacterial infection of their tarsals that is difficult to treat. Many of the organisms causing OM are opportunistic pathogens taking advantage of the poor immune response in the host or accidental placement into a site, which overcomes the normal barriers to an infection.

Our patient has OM caused by *P. aeruginosa*, which has multiple virulence factors that enable it to be a very effective opportunistic pathogen. Some of these virulence factors are common to all gram-negative rods, such as presence of a capsule, pili, and lipopolysaccharide. Other virulence factors are unique to *P. aeruginosa*, such as the production of pyocyanin pigment that inhibits the beating of the ciliated cells in the upper airway and allows bacteria to journey into the lower respiratory tract. *P. aeruginosa* produces several exotoxins (exotoxins A and S) that inhibit protein synthesis in host cells by ADP ribosylating elongation factor 2. Exotoxin A, the most important factor for virulence, has the same functional activity as does diphtheria exotoxin, but its structure and receptors on the host cell are different. Exotoxin S is toxic to neutrophils, while exotoxin U kills macrophages. Two enzymes, LasA and LasB, destroy elastin-containing tissues in the lung and blood vessels. Without elastin, the alveoli can no longer expand and contract with air intake and release, and blood vessels are no longer pliant and can rupture, causing hemorrhagic lesions in the skin (ecthyma gangrenosum) (Fig. 8.8).

The capsule of *P. aeruginosa* is composed of an exopolysaccharide (alginate) that anchors the organism to the epithelial cells. Dense layers of these bacteria accumulate in this polysaccharide matrix, forming a biofilm on catheters and plastic implants. The bacteria in a biofilm are less susceptible to antibiotics than free-living bacteria, and they are protected from the phagocytic activity of the host cells. Strains of *P. aeruginosa* producing copious amounts of alginate appear as very mucoid colonies on the culture plates, and these are most often observed in the respiratory cultures of patients with cystic fibrosis who are colonized by these strains. The principle virulence factors for *P. aeruginosa* are listed in Table 8.2.

The breath of virulence factors helps explain the diversity of diseases caused by *P. aeruginosa*. Because this organism has minimal nutritional

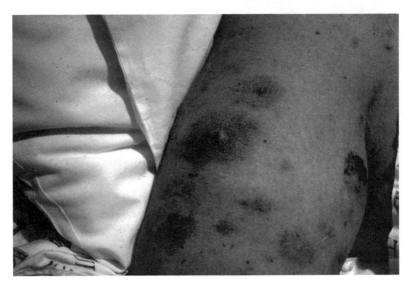

FIGURE 8.8 Ecthyma gangrenosum.

TABLE 8.2.	Virulence Factors of *P. aeruginosa* and Their Mechanisms of Action
Virulence Factor	**Mechanisms of Action**
Capsule	Anchors bacterial cells to host epithelial cells Protects organism from phagocytic activity Protects organism from antibiotic activity
Pili	Adherence to host epithelial cells
Adhesin	Non-pilus-related, adherence to chloride channel protein in lung and eye
Lipopolysaccharide	Endotoxin mediating septic shock
Phospholipase C	Hemolysin that breaks down lipids and lecithin
Pyocyanin	Impairs motility of cilia Mediates tissue damage
Exotoxin A	Required for virulence Inhibits protein synthesis similar to diphtheria toxin Causes tissue damage in lung, cornea, wounds
Exotoxin S	Inhibits protein synthesis Toxic for PMNs
Exotoxin U	Toxic for macrophages
Elastase	Enzymes destroy elastin in lung and blood vessels Inhibits neutrophil chemotaxis Degrades complement

requirements, it can grow in a diversity of moist environments such as tap water, pond water, and other moist environments. *P. aeruginosa* is a well-known cause of nosocomial infections. Live plants and flowers are not allowed in intensive care units since this microorganism can grow well in these environments and be transmitted to immunocompromised patients. Swimmer's ear (otitis externa) and folliculitis are acquired from swimming pools, hot tubs, and whirlpools with high colony counts of *Pseudomonas*. Corneal ulcers can result from pseudomonal infection from contaminated contact lens solutions or abrasions. Ventilator-associated pneumonia and urinary tract infections occur in patients who have biofilms forming in their life-saving devices.

Pseudomonas is a major threat to patients in burn units whose primary defense against infection is now gone. Biopsy cultures of the skin alert the physicians when to perform extensive debridement to remove tissue with high colony counts of *P. aeruginosa*. OM occurs in patients following trauma in a wet environment. Water-related accidents or puncture wounds through a moist sneaker sole allow this opportunistic pathogen easy entry into deeper tissues, where it can destroy host cells and break down tissues.

Pseudomonas bacteremia occurs in patients with hematologic malignancies, diabetes mellitus, and burns. *Pseudomonas* endocarditis occurs in intravenous drug users who inject their drugs with contaminated syringes. *P. aeruginosa* is most commonly associated with individuals who have cystic fibrosis (CF). The organism colonizes the respiratory tract, and the prolific production of alginate capsule makes it difficult to clear these secretions from the upper airways of CF patients. Multiple courses of antibiotics lead to colonization with antimicrobial-resistant strains of *P. aeruginosa* that cause breathing problems for those with this disease, many of whom go on to require a lung transplant for survival.

8.6. TREATMENT AND PREVENTION

Plain x-rays, bone scan, CT scan, and magnetic resonance imaging (MRI) may all be helpful in the diagnosis of OM. However, it is imperative to obtain a culture of the material by either percutaneous aspirate or surgical procedure before beginning antimicrobial therapy. The optimal length of treatment is unknown, but the total duration of parenteral therapy for OM is usually 4–6 weeks. The infection must be treated aggressively to eradicate all viable bacteria to prevent a chronic infection. In chronic OM, surgical removal of dead bone tissue is usually required. Antibiotic therapy without surgical debridement is not likely to be curative in chronic OM. The open space left by the removed bone tissue can be filled with bone graft or packing material to promote the growth of new bone tissue. Infection involving an orthopedic prosthesis may require surgical removal of the prosthesis and of the infected tissue surrounding the area. The outcome is usually good with adequate treatment of acute OM. The prognosis is frequently poor for chronic OM, even with surgery. Resistant chronic OM may result in amputation, particularly in diabetics or other patients with poor blood circulation.

TABLE 8.3.	Nonenteric Gram-Negative Bacteria and Their Medical Importance	
Organisms	Gram Stain	Characteristics
Stenotrophomonas maltophilia	Gram-negative rod	Formerly called *Pseudomonas maltophilia* Found in moist environments Causes nosocomial infections Resistant to commonly prescribed antibiotics
Burkholderia cepacia	Gram-negative rod	Formerly called *Pseudomonas cepacia* Found in moist environments Serious pathogen for patients with CF Resistant to many antibiotics and disinfectants
Aeromonas species	Gram-negative rod	Found in aquatic environments Causes gastroenteritis and wound infections
Acinetobacter species	Gram-negative coccobacillus	Found in moist environments Causes serious nosocomial infections in respiratory tract, wounds, and bloodstream Some strains are resistant to all commonly used antibiotics
Legionella pneumophila	Small gram-negative rod	Found in air conditioners, hot tubs, humidifiers, water pipes Causes nosocomial and community-acquired pneumonia Requires specialized media to grow in culture Resistant to β-lactam antibiotics

P. aeruginosa is intrinsically resistant to many of the commonly prescribed antibiotics, such as ampicillin, first- and second-generation cephalosporins, trimethoprim–sulfamethoxazole, macrolides (erythromycin, clarithromycin), and tetracycline. Therapy with an extended-spectrum β-lactam (ticarcillin, piperacillin) or third-generation cephalosporin (ceftazidime) or a fluoroquinolone (levofloxacin, ciprofloxacin) is needed to treat a systemic infection with this organism. Sometimes an aminoglycoside (gentamicin, tobramycin, amikacin) is added as well. These versatile bacteria have many ways to become resistant to antimicrobial agents. They can alter the size and shape of their porins, the holes where the drug must enter. They have efflux pumps to remove an antibiotic before it reaches its target, and they can degrade an antibiotic with enzymes. Fluoroquinolones (ciprofloxacin) are the only class of antibiotics with activity against *Pseudomonas* that can be given orally.

8.7. ADDITIONAL POINTS

■ Prior to the availability of a vaccine, 5–10% of cases of pediatric OM were caused by *Haemophilus influenzae* type b. With routine immunization of children, this organism has disappeared as an invasive pathogen. Care should be taken to document immunization with *H. influenzae* vaccine before selecting empiric antibiotic therapy.

■ Determination of CRP is a simple way of measuring the degree of the inflammatory response. Studies have shown that a high CRP after three days of antibiotic treatment for OM is associated with short-term adverse outcome and the development of radiographic changes in children.

■ Tuberculous OM may occur in any bone, including the ribs, skull, phalanx, pelvis, and the spine, where the infection may involve multiple vertebrae and extend into the soft-tissue-forming abscesses (Pott's disease). In patients who are at risk for an extrapulmonary manifestation of tuberculosis, a tuberculin skin test (PPD) should be placed, and an acid-fast stain should be performed on any specimens sent to pathology and microbiology labs. Because very few organisms may be present in the pus, molecular tests may be required to make the diagnosis since cultures are often negative.

■ Other medically important nonenteric gram-negative rods are listed in Table 8.3.

SUGGESTED READING

CALHOUN, J. H. AND M. M. MANRING, Adult osteomyelitis, *Infect. Dis. Clin. N. Am.* **19**: 765–786 (2005).

KAPLAN, S. L., Osteomyelitis in children, *Infect. Dis. Clin. N. Am.* **19**: 787–797 (2005).

Salyers, A. A. AND D. D. Whitt, *Bacterial Pathogenesis: A Molecular Approach*, 2nd ed., ASM Press, Washington, DC, 2002, pp. 247–262.

TRAUTMANN, M., P. M. LEPPER, AND M. HALLER, Ecology of *Pseudomonas aeruginosa* in the intensive care unit and the evolving role of water outlets as a reservoir for the organism, *Am. J. Infect. Control* **33**: S41–S49 (2005).

Woman with Acute Abdominal Pain and Cervical Discharge

9.1. PATIENT HISTORY

A 20 year-old female college student presents with 3 days of vague lower abdominal discomfort, mild dysuria, and urinary frequency. A urinalysis, done by her family internist, revealed 50 WBCs and no RBCs. Gram stain and culture of the urine were negative. She now presents to student health with the same symptoms and describes vaginal itching with a yellowish vaginal discharge. She has no history of medical problems. She tested negative for human immunodeficiency virus (HIV) 6 months ago. She has had a new male sexual partner for the past week, and had three other male partners during the past year. She denies use of tobacco, alcohol, or intravenous drugs. Her only medication is oral contraceptives. On examination, she is well-appearing, afebrile, with normal vital signs. The physical exam is entirely normal with the exception of the pelvic exam. The cervical mucosa is edematous and friable, and there is a mucopurulent cervical discharge. There is no significant pain on cervical motion, or palpation of the ovaries. A pregnancy test was negative.

Medical Microbiology for the New Curriculum: A Case-Based Approach, by Roberta B. Carey, Mindy G. Schuster, and Karin L. McGowan.
Copyright © 2008 John Wiley & Sons, Inc.

9.2. DIFFERENTIAL DIAGNOSIS

Infectious Causes

Bacteria

Chlamydia trachomatis

Gardnerella vaginalis (bacterial vaginosis)

Neisseria gonorrhoeae

Treponema pallidum (syphilis)

Viruses

Herpes simplex virus (HSV)

Fungi

Candida spp.

Parasites

Trichomonas vaginalis

Noninfectious Causes

Cervical or vaginal malignancies

Chemical/allergic vulvovaginitis (from douche or spermacide)

CLINICAL CLUES

? Presence of genital lesions? Genital ulcers are most commonly caused by herpes simplex virus.

? Presence of genital warts? These are most often caused by human papilloma virus (HPV).

? Presence of vaginal discharge? Characteristics of vaginal discharge are not particularly helpful diagnostically, as there is much overlap with different etiologies.

9.3. LABORATORY TESTS

Sexually transmitted diseases (STDs) can present as a wide spectrum of illnesses, including general urethritis or cervicitis, vaginal discharge, genital ulcers, genital warts, swelling and inflammation of the epididymis (epididymitis), and pelvic inflammatory disease (PID). In addition, with those who practice receptive anal intercourse, gastrointestinal syndromes of diarrhea and abdominal cramping (enteritis), rectal inflammation (proctitis), and rectal and colonic inflammation (proctocolitis) may also be indicators of an STD. *Chlamydia trachomatis* and *Neisseria gonorrhoeae* are the two most common causes of STD in the United States. For this reason, initial screening for both pathogens is recommended. If genital ulcers are present, one should order a test for HSV and a syphilis screening test because a dual infection is possible.

A wide range of testing methods is presently available for the laboratory diagnosis of *C. trachomatis* and *N. gonorrhoeae*. They include the nucleic acid amplification test (NAAT), nucleic acid probe, immunoassay (EIA), direct fluorescent antibody (DFA) for *C. trachomatis*, Gram stain for *N. gonorrhoeae*, and culture for both organisms. NAAT tests for both *N. gonorrhoeae* and *C. trachomatis* are more sensitive than nonamplification assays and are now the method of choice in many laboratories. The same specimen (endocervical swab, urethral swab, or urine) can be used to test for both organisms simultaneously, turnaround time is shorter, and large numbers of specimens can be batch-tested. Rectal swabs, pharyngeal swabs, and specimens from cases of suspected sexual assault and/or sexual abuse may not be tested using NAAT. Culture is the recommended method of choice in these cases for both agents.

The specific test used for screening for an STD usually dictates the type of specimen that should be taken. For a NAAT screening for *C. trachomatis* and/or *N. gonorrhoeae*, endocervical and urethral swabs or urine can be submitted from women and urethral swabs or urine can be submitted from males. Specimens obtained for NAAT should be obtained and transported as directed by each test kit manufacturer using swabs and transport media supplied by the manufacturer.

For non-NAAT or culture for both *C. trachomatis* and *N. gonorrhoeae*, the specimen of choice is an endocervical or urethral swab. To obtain a urethral specimen, a specially designed rayon, Dacron, or cotton-tipped swab is inserted approximately 2 cm into the urethra and gently rotated in one direction and then removed. Even if urethral discharge is present, it is critical to remove epithelial cells because *C. trachomatis* is an intracellular organism and discharge alone is not sufficient. To obtain an endocervical specimen, a large swab should be used to remove all secretions and discharge from the cervical os. Then a specially designed rayon, Dacron, or cotton-tipped swab should be inserted 1–2 cm into the endocervical canal and rotated against the wall of the canal for at least 30 s before removal. When screening men or women with possible rectal or pharyngeal infections, rectal or pharyngeal swab specimens should be submitted specifically for culture for *N. gonorrhoeae*, and both culture and DFA for *C. trachomatis*.

In males who have urethral exudate, a definitive diagnosis of gonorrhea can be achieved by finding intracellular (within polymorphonuclear neutrophils) gram negative diplococci with flattened adjacent sides on a Gram stain of the discharge (Fig. 9.1). Gram stain cannot be used to diagnose gonorrhea in women because a number of organisms that represent normal vaginal flora can give results that resemble those seen with *N. gonorrhoeae*.

Careful attention must be paid to maintain the viability of both *C. trachomatis* and *N. gonorrhoeae* during transport to a laboratory. Swabs for *C. trachomatis* culture are best transported in specific transport media containing antibiotics. If transport time will be ≤24 h, the sample should be stored at 4°C. If samples cannot be processed in ≤24 h, they should be frozen at -70°C. Specimens submitted for *N. gonorrhoeae* culture should be

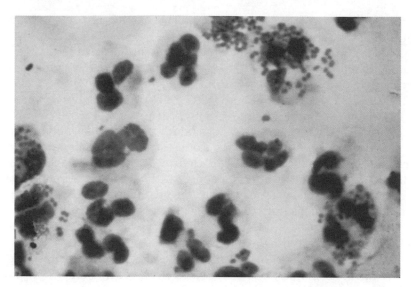

FIGURE 9.1 Gram stain showing intra- and extracellular gram-negative diplococci.

inoculated directly onto a chocolate-based selective medium (e.g., Thayer-Martin, Martin-Lewis, New York City medium) and immediately placed in a CO_2-enriched atmosphere. For transport to a reference lab, specimens should be directly inoculated in a W pattern onto a self-contained commercial transport medium such as JEMBEC or Transgrow, both of which generate their own CO_2 atmosphere using a sodium bicarbonate tablet (Fig. 9.2). Once received in the laboratory, the inoculated culture medium is incubated at 35°C in 5–8% CO_2. Plates are examined daily and held for a

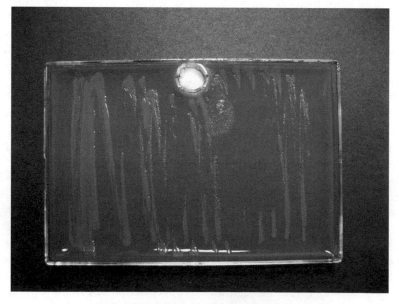

FIGURE 9.2 Inoculated Jembec agar.

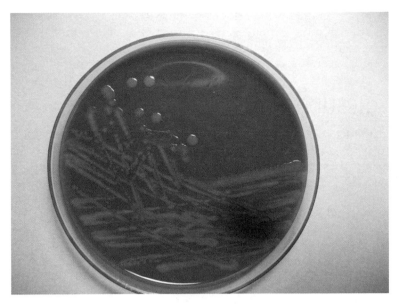

FIGURE 9.3 *Neisseria gonorrhoeae* colonies an Thayer–Martin agar.

total of 72 h before discarding. Colonies of N. *gonorrhoeae* are grayish-white and shiny in appearance and are oxidase-positive (Fig. 9.3). All oxidase-positive gram-negative diplococci are presumptive *Neisseria* or *Moraxella* spp. and must be further tested to be confirmed as N. *gonorrhoeae*. Methods used to achieve confirmation include acid production from carbohydrate testing and nucleic acid probes. N. *gonorrhoeae* is positive for acid production in glucose but negative for sucrose, lactose, and maltose (Fig. 9.4).

While standard methods for performing antimicrobial susceptibility testing have been established for N. *gonorrhoeae*, routine testing of isolates is seldom performed because treatment guidelines for STDs are routinely published by the Centers for Disease Control and Prevention (CDC).

Serology is unhelpful in diagnosing *Chlamydia* infections since antibody titers persist, and it is impossible to distinguish a current infection

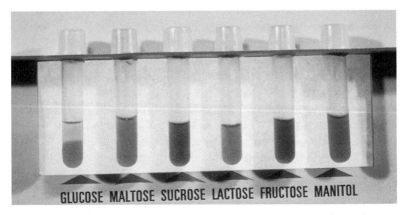

FIGURE 9.4 Carbohydrate fermentation tests (positive glucose).

from a previous one. No serological test exists for *N. gonorrhoeae*. Since urine culture and urine analysis have already been performed on this patient, screening tests for both *C. trachomatis* and *N. gonorrhoeae* should be performed. An endocervical swab was obtained and submitted for NAAT.

9.4. RESULTS

This patient's endocervical specimen was positive for both *C. trachomatis* and *N. gonorrhoeae* by NAAT. All positive screening tests should be considered presumptive evidence of infection. The requirements for reporting STDs differ by state, but clinicians are expected to be familiar with the requirements in their local areas. At this time, syphilis, gonorrhea, chlamydia, and HIV are reportable infections in every state.

9.5. PATHOGENESIS

C. trachomatis occurs worldwide and is the most commonly reported sexually transmitted disease in the United States, with the highest rates occurring in young females 16–24 years of age. Transmission occurs silently from person to person since the infection can be asymptomatic in 80% of the infected women and 25% of infected men. Infection does not confer long-lasting immunity, and reinfection causes a vigorous inflammatory response and tissue damage.

C. trachomatis has two morphological forms: the small infectious form, known as the elementary body (EB), and the larger replicative form, known as the reticulate body (RB). Infection occurs according to the cycle shown in Fig. 9.5.

N. gonorrhoeae is the second most commonly reported STD in the United States. Gonorrhea is a major global health problem with more than 60 million cases each year in the world. Although *N. gonorrhoeae* may be difficult to grow in the laboratory, it is easily transmitted from person to person because it is attached to sperm. Humans are the only reservoir for this microorganism, and patients may be asymptomatic, similar to what occurs with chlamydial infections. The risk of infection increases with multiple sexual partners. The peak incidence of infection occurs in 15–24 year-olds.

N. gonorrhoeae has multiple virulence factors that can affect the infectious cycle. Pili are critical structures for infection, and cells without pili are avirulent. Pili mediate attachment to the nonciliated epithelial cells and provide resistance to killing by neutrophils. Antigenic variation occurs on pilin proteins, which leads to a lack of protective immunity. Opacity proteins (opa) mediate a tighter binding to the host cells and facilitate adherence of the bacterial cells to one another. Porin proteins (por) protect the bacteria from intracellular killing by preventing phagolysosome fusion in the neutrophil, thus allowing the organisms to survive. Lipooligosaccharide (LOS) is the major antigen in the cell wall, similar to lipopolysaccharide (LPS) in other gram-negative organisms. LOS has endotoxin activity and stimulates host inflammatory response and release of tumor necrosis factor (TNFα). Antibody directed to the pili, opa, and

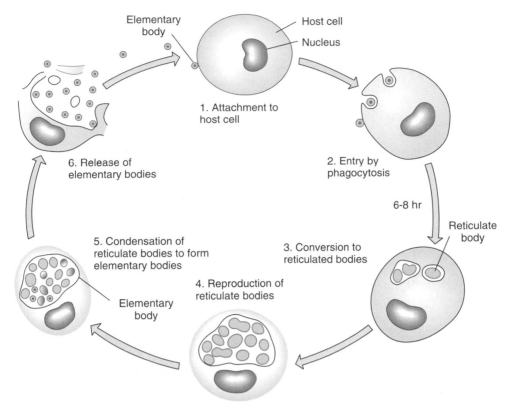

FIGURE 9.5 Infectious cycle of *Chlamydia trachomatis*.

por proteins can inhibit further multiplication of the bacteria. Antibody produced to LOS activates complement and controls the infection. The infectious cycle for *N. gonorrhoeae* is described in Fig. 9.6. Three sites where antibody can interrupt the cycle of infection are at the points where opa, por, and LOS interact with the host cells.

In females the gonococci can ascend from the cervix into the uterus and enter the fallopian tubes, causing an infection known as salpingitis, or pelvic inflammatory disease (PID). Early diagnosis and prompt treatment are necessary to prevent irreversible damage to the fallopian tubes, which results in infertility. In 1% of the cases, the infection can disseminate to the joints (arthritis), the heart (endocarditis), or central nervous system (meningitis). *N. gonorrhoeae* can also infect the oral and rectal mucosa. Chlamydial infection can also cause infertility.

9.6. TREATMENT AND PREVENTION

Because of the difference in structure between *C. trachomatis* and *N. gonorrhoeae*, no single antibiotic is effective against both microorganisms. A macrolide, such as azithromycin, or doxycycline may be prescribed for a genital chlamydial infection. Azithromycin can be given as a single dose and this may be preferable to a seven day course of doxycycline if patient

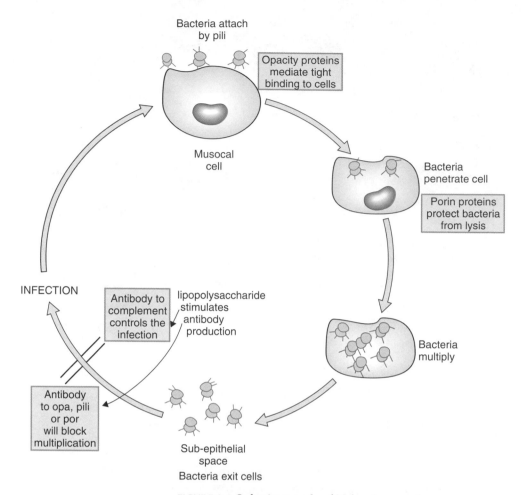

FIGURE 9.6 Infectious cycle of *Neisseria gonorrhoeae*.

compliance is a concern. β-Lactams are not effective. For the treatment of uncomplicated gonococcal infections of the cervix, urethra, and rectum, the CDC recommends a single IM dose of ceftriaxone or a single oral dose of cefixime. CDC no longer recommends the use of fluoroquinolones (ciprofloxacin, levofloxacin or ofloxacin) for the treatment of gonococcal infection and associated conditions such as pelvic inflammatory disease because of increasing resistance, especially among men who have sex with men. Penicillin is no longer the drug of choice, due to the presence of β-lactamase and chromosome-mediated resistance. The CDC publishes guidelines based on antimicrobial susceptibility data gathered from state public health laboratories to issue warnings of changes in antibiotic susceptibility for particular regions of the country. Recurrent STDs are more often due to reinfection than treatment failure. It is important to notify and treat the sexual partners.

To prevent gonococcal eye infection, chemoprophylaxis of newborns includes administration of silver nitrate drops or erythromycin or tetracycline ointment. Treatment of newborns with pneumonia or conjunctivitis caused by *C. trachomatis* is usually a course of erythromycin. Currently there is no vaccine to prevent infection with either of these pathogens.

9.7. ADDITIONAL POINTS

■ The systemic disease syphilis is caused by *Treponema pallidum*, an organism that cannot be cultured in vitro. Laboratory diagnosis can be made by the microscopic identification of *T. pallidum* in clinical specimens (darkfield exam or direct fluorescent antibody) or by serology tests that are classified as either nontreponemal or treponemal. Nontreponemal tests are nonspecific and measure anticardiolipin antibodies. The most commonly used nontreponemal tests are the rapid plasma reagin (RPR) and the Venereal Disease Research Laboratory (VDRL) tests. Both can be performed using serum; however, only the VDRL test can be used for testing CSF. Nontreponemal antibody results are reported quantitatively (1 : 4, 1 : 8, 1 : 16, etc.), and the level of titer usually corresponds to the level of disease. As patients are successfully treated, the titer will go down. While nontreponemal tests are excellent screening tests, all positives must be confirmed with a more specific treponemal test because of false-positive reactions associated with other systemic and autoimmune diseases.

■ The most commonly used specific treponemal tests are the fluorescent treponemal antibody absorption (FTA-ABS) and the microhemagglutination assay (MHA). Both are recommended as confirmatory tests and as tests for diagnosing very early or late syphilis when nontreponemal tests have not yet become reactive or may have reverted to negative. Because treponemal tests remain reactive for many years after effective treatment, they cannot be used to follow a treatment course.

■ Bacterial vaginosis (BV) is a disease characterized by a vaginal discharge and a replacement of the normal vaginal flora with high concentrations of anaerobic bacteria (*Prevotella* spp., *Bacteroides* spp., *Mobiluncus* spp.), *Mycoplasma hominis,* and *Gardnerella vaginalis*. A clinical diagnosis of BV is made when three of the following four criteria are observed:

1. The presence of a homogeneous discharge that adheres to the walls of the vagina

2. The presence of clue cells—these are large squamous epithelial cells with gram-variable coccobacilli and rods attached to their surfaces

3. A pH of vaginal fluid of >4.5

4. A fishy amine odor of the vaginal discharge before or after the addition of 10% KOH (this is called the "whiff test").

■ A Gram stain can be used to observe clue cells and to score the bacterial morphologies characteristic of BV (Nugent score). A DNA probe-based test (Affirm™) is also available for detecting high concentrations of *G. vaginalis* resulting from the shift in normal vaginal flora.

■ *Haemophilus ducreyi* is the cause of a genital ulcer disease called chancroid. Like other *Haemophilus* spp., *H. ducreyi* is a fastidious gram-negative rod. At this time, the gold standard for the laboratory diagnosis is growing *H. ducreyi* in culture; however, even with the use of special chocolate agar–based culture media, the sensitivity of culture is ≤80%. A number of PCR assays have been developed for the diagnosis of *H. ducreyi* as well as the other agents causing genital ulcers (*T. pallidum*, HSV-1, HSV-2), but at the present time, there is no FDA-approved PCR test for *H. ducreyi* in the United States.

■ Testing for HIV should be offered to all patients seen and evaluated for STDs; however, informed consent (sometimes written) is required before such testing can be performed. Initial testing for HIV makes use of sensitive screening tests for antibodies to HIV-1/2. A positive antibody screening test must be confirmed by more specific tests such as Western blot or an immunofluorescence assay. A negative HIV-1/2 antibody screening test usually indicates that a person is not infected unless the infection has been recently acquired (within 3 months). Refer to Case 24 for additional testing information.

SUGGESTED READING

CDC, Screening tests to detect *Chlamydia trachomatis* and *Neisseria gonorrhoeae* infections—2002, *MMWR* **51** (RR-15):1–38 (2002).

CDC, Sexually transmitted diseases treatment guidelines: 2006, *MMWR* **55** (RR-11):1–94 (2006).

CDC. Update to CDC's sexually transmitted diseases treatment guidelines, 2006: fluoroquinolones no longer recommended for treatment of gonococcal infections. *MMWR* **56**:332–336.

EDWARDS, J. L. AND M. A. APICELLA, The molecular mechanisms used by *Neisseria gonorrhoeae* to initiate infection differ between men and women, *Clin. Microbiol. Rev.* **17**:965–981 (2004).

OLSHEN, E. AND L. A. SHRIER, Diagnostics tests for chlamydial and gonorrheal infections, *Semin. Pediatr. Infect. Dis.* **16**:192–198 (2005).

Woman with Acute Fever and Productive Cough

10.1. PATIENT HISTORY

A previously healthy 67 year-old woman is seen in the emergency department (ED) with the chief complaint of abrupt onset of fever, chills, productive cough of yellow sputum, and shortness of breath of 3 days' duration. Her son brought her to the hospital when she became slightly disoriented. Her past medical history was unremarkable. She lives alone in her own home, has no pets, is presently taking no medications, and does not smoke. While she has not traveled outside her rural town in Delaware for years, her two grandchildren ages 5 and 6 years have been staying with her for the past 2 weeks prior to the start of their school year. When questioned, she reported she had not been vaccinated "for anything" in the past 10 years. On physical exam (PE) she appeared uncomfortable and short of breath. Her temperature was 40°C (104°F). Her respiratory rate was 34 breaths/min, heart rate 140 beats/min, and blood pressure 94/50 mm Hg. There was no lymphadenopathy. Chest exam revealed crackles (rales) at both lung bases. She was lethargic, but oriented to place and time. The remainder of her PE was within normal limits.

10.2. DIFFERENTIAL DIAGNOSIS

This patient's acute onset, fever, productive cough, and shortness of breath suggest a lower respiratory tract infection, in particular, pneumonia. Other

Medical Microbiology for the New Curriculum: A Case-Based Approach, by Roberta B. Carey, Mindy G. Schuster, and Karin L. McGowan.
Copyright © 2008 John Wiley & Sons, Inc.

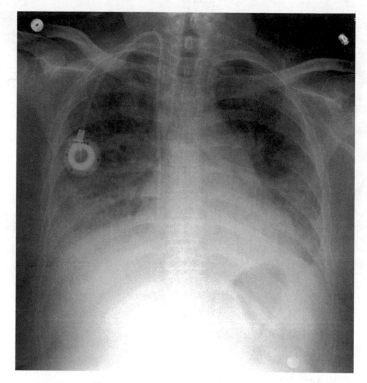

FIGURE 10.1 Chest x-ray showing bilateral lobar pneumonia.

possibilities include bronchitis, empyema, lung abscess, lung cancer, and sarcoid. All patients suspected of having pneumonia should receive a chest x-ray promptly as this is a critical test for establishing the diagnosis of pneumonia and distinguishing it from bronchitis. While in the ED, this patient received a chest x-ray, which showed infiltrates localized in the lower lobes of both lungs (bilateral lobar pneumonia) (Fig. 10.1). This confirmed the diagnosis of pneumonia. Pneumonia is further characterized as being community-acquired, hospital-acquired (nosocomial) pneumonia, aspiration pneumonia, or pneumonia in an immunocompromised patient. It is important to establish the type of pneumonia because the etiology of each type can differ significantly. Because she is a normal host, living at home with no chronic illness, this patient has community-acquired pneumonia (CAP).

Infectious Causes

Organisms responsible for causing CAP in immunocompetent adults include those listed below.

Bacteria

Chlamydia pneumoniae

Haemophilus influenzae

Legionella pneumophila

Mycoplasma pneumoniae

Staphylococcus aureus — uncommon cause of CAP, usually seen as a superinfection following an initial lung infection with influenza virus

Streptococcus pneumoniae — the most common cause of CAP

Rare causes: *Streptococcus pyogenes, Neisseria meningitidis, Moraxella catarrhalis, Klebsiella pneumoniae* and other gram-negative rods, *Chlamydia psittaci, Coxiella burnetii, and Francisella tularensis*

Fungi

Blastomyces dermatitidis

Coccidioides immitis

Cryptococcus neoformans

Histoplasma capsulatum

Parasites

Parasites are not a cause of community-acquired pneumonia.

Viruses

Adenovirus

Corona virus [severe acute respiratory syndrome (SARS)]

Influenza virus

Parainfluenza virus

Respiratory syncytial virus

Risk Factors

While a large number of organisms can cause CAP, most cases are caused by only a few; the major pathogen is *S. pneumoniae*. A patient's age, living conditions, geographic location, travel history, attendance in daycare or a nursing home, season of the year, and exposures to environmental conditions or animals can all be risk factors for specific pathogens. Once again, a well-taken history is critical if one hopes to detect unusual causes of pneumonia. Risk factors and epidemiologic associations that are well known for organisms causing CAP in immunocompetent as well as immunocompromised hosts are listed in Table 10.1.

CLINICAL CLUES

[?] Presence of pleural effusion? Common in patients with pneumococcal and mycoplasma pneumonia, and many patients will have associated chest pain. The effusion is most often inflammatory (parapneumonic), rather than infectious (empyema).

[?] Recent influenza infection? Pneumococcal pneumonia is the most common secondary infection following influenza.

[?] Is this a patient with "atypical" pneumonia (*Legionella, Mycoplasma, Chlamydia*)? It is not possible to differentiate pneumococcal from atypical pneumonia by physical exam or chest x-ray.

TABLE 10.1.	Possible Etiologic Agents Causing Pneumonia Based on Risk Factors	

Risk Factor/Condition	Possible Etiologic Agents
Environmental exposures	
Exposure to birds	*Chlamydia psittaci*
Exposure to bats or bird feces–enriched soil	*Histoplasma capsulatum*
Exposure to community with active influenza	Influenza, *Streptococcus pneumoniae, Staphylococcus aureus, Streptococcus pyogenes, Haemophilus influenzae*
Exposure to contaminated air-conditioning cooling towers; grocery store mist machines; recent stay in hotel or hospital; hot tub	*Legionella* spp.
Exposure to mice or mice droppings	Hantavirus
Exposure to parturient cats or farm animals	*Coxiella burnetii*
Exposure to pneumonia outbreak in military training camp	*Streptococcus pneumoniae, Chlamydia pneumoniae, Mycoplasma pneumoniae,* adenovirus
Exposure to pneumonia outbreak in jail or homeless shelter	*Streptococcus pneumoniae, Mycobacterium tuberculosis*
Exposure to pneumonia in nursing home	*Streptococcus pneumoniae, Chlamydia pneumoniae,* influenza A virus, respiratory syncytial virus
Exposure to rabbits	*Francisella tularensis, Yersinia pestis*
Host factors	
Alcoholism	*Streptococcus pneumoniae,* anaerobes, *Staphylococcus aureus, Klebsiella pneumoniae*
Aspiration event	Anaerobes, *Streptococcus pneumoniae, Haemophilus influenzae, Staphylococcus aureus*
B-cell defects (e.g., Hodgkin's disease, multiple myeloma)	*Streptococcus pneumoniae*
Chronic obstructive pulmonary disease	*Streptococcus pneumoniae, Haemophilus influenzae, Moraxella catarrhalis, Legionella* spp.
Poor dental hygiene	Anaerobes
Diabetic ketoacidosis	*Streptococcus pneumoniae, Staphylococcus aureus*

TABLE 10.1.	(Continued)
Risk Factor/Condition	**Possible Etiologic Agents**
Granulocytopenia	*Escherichia coli, Klebsiella pneumoniae*, and other aerobic gram-negative rods
Healthcare worker	*Mycobacterium tuberculosis*
HIV infection (early)	*Streptococcus pneumoniae, Haemophilus influenzae, Mycobacterium tuberculosis*
HIV infection CD4 count <200/μL	*Pneumocystis carinii, Cryptococcus neoformans, Streptococcus pneumoniae, Haemophilus influenzae, Histoplasma capsulatum, Mycobacterium tuberculosis, Rhodococcus equi*
Injection drug use	*Staphylococcus aureus, Streptococcus pneumoniae*, anaerobes, *Mycobacterium tuberculosis*
Nursing home residency	*Streptococcus pneumoniae, Haemophilus influenzae, Staphylococcus aureus, Chlamydia pneumoniae*, anaerobes, gram-negative rods
Sickle cell disease	*Streptococcus pneumoniae*
Smoking	*Streptococcus pneumoniae, Haemophilus influenzae, Moraxella catarrhalis, Legionella* spp.
Solid-organ transplantation (≥ 90 days post - transplant)	*Streptococcus pneumoniae, Haemophilus influenzae, Legionella* spp., *Pneumocystis carinii*, cytomegalovirus, *Strongyloides stercoralis*
Structural lung disease (e.g., cystic fibrosis)	*Pseudomonas aeruginosa, Staphylococcus aureus, Burkholderia cepacia*
Travel	
Travel to southwestern USA or massive sand exposure in same endemic zone	*Coccidioides immitis*
Travel to Mississippi and Ohio River valleys, New York State, or exposure to excavation in same endemic zone	*Histoplasma capsulatum*
Travel to Southeast Asia, Thailand or China	*Burkholderia pseudomallei, Penicillium marnefeii*, severe acute respiratory syndrome (SARS)
Travel to countries with high incidence of tuberculosis	*Mycobacterium tuberculosis*

10.3. LABORATORY TESTS

Guidelines for the management of CAP recommend that all patients suspected of having pneumonia receive a chest x-ray. In addition, in patients who have positive x-rays and are admitted because of age (>50 years) or other comorbid conditions such as congestive heart failure or neoplastic, hepatic, renal, or cerebrovascular disease, the following laboratory tests should be performed: complete blood count (CBC) and differential, serum creatinine, blood urea nitrogen, glucose, electrolytes, oxygen saturation testing, and liver function tests.

Two pretreatment sets of blood cultures as well as a Gram stain and culture of pretreatment expectorated sputum should be submitted for routine bacterial culture. Human immunodeficiency virus (HIV) serology for persons aged 15–54 years should also be considered (with informed consent) because the list of possible etiologic agents that are treatable would dramatically change if a patient were HIV serology positive. If present, pleural fluid should be submitted for Gram stain and bacterial culture. Testing should also be performed in patients with the appropriate environmental exposures or host risks to rule out tuberculosis and *Legionella* infection (see Section 10.7). Additional microbiology testing should be considered only if clinical features, underlying conditions, season of the year, epidemiologic exposures, host factors, or travel history obtained from a carefully taken history and physical exam warrant testing for specific agents.

For collection of sputum, patients should be instructed to rinse or gargle with water to remove debris and contaminating oral flora before coughing a deep specimen into a sterile, screwcapped container. When patients are unable to produce sputum (infants, children, the elderly), a sample can be collected using suction. The specimen should be transported to the laboratory at room temperature. Ideally, specimens should be transported to the lab within 2 h.

The purpose of sputum Gram stain is twofold: to assess the quality of the sputum specimen obtained and to identify a specific etiologic agent(s). A variety of grading systems are available for evaluating sputum quality, but in general, an adequate specimen is one that yields >25 polymorphonuclear neutrophils (PMNs) and <10 squamous epithelial cells per low-power field (Fig. 10.2). Specimens not meeting these criteria are considered saliva and should not be further processed for culture (Fig. 10.3). Sputum specimens considered adequate for culture are plated onto 5% sheep blood agar, chocolate agar, and MacConkey agar. Sputum is not processed for anaerobic culture because, when expectorated, it passes through the mouth, which contains normal anaerobic flora.

For patients with CAP who cannot produce sputum, or have a nondiagnostic sputum Gram stain, testing for *Legionella pneumophila* urine antigen should be considered.

10.4. LABORATORY RESULTS

The Gram stain of the patient's sputum specimen showed many WBCs and moderate gram-positive cocci in pairs and chains. Because only WBCs

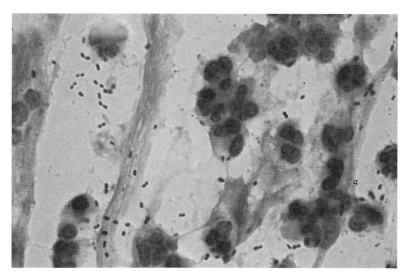

FIGURE 10.2 Sputum Gram stain showing acceptable specimen quality.

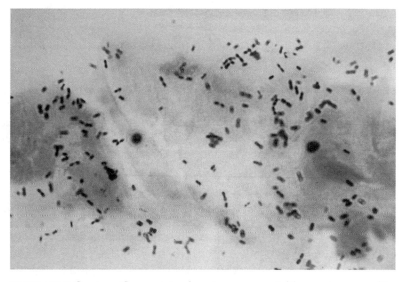

FIGURE 10.3 Sputum Gram stain showing unacceptable specimen quality.

and no squamous epithelial cells were seen, the specimen was considered adequate. Even more significant is the fact that only one morphological type of bacteria was seen on the smear, meaning that this organism is probably causing the pneumonia. Morphologically, *S. pneumoniae* (also called pneumococci) appears as gram-positive cocci in chains and pairs, which are frequently called "lancet-shaped" diplococci because the distal ends of the paired cells tend to be pointed (Fig. 10.4). Both the blood and sputum cultures grew *S. pneumoniae*, which appears as an α-hemolytic (greening of medium) colonies on blood agar. Because of its capsule, the organism may also appear mucoid. *S. pneumoniae* can be differentiated from other α-hemolytic streptococci that are normal

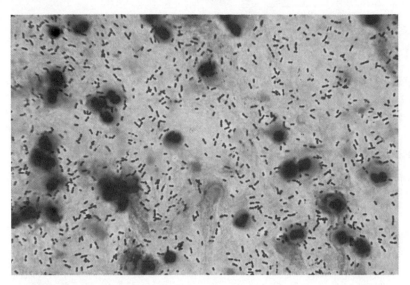

FIGURE 10.4 Sputum Gram stain showing WBCs and lancet- shaped gram-positive diplococci.

upper respiratory flora (called viridans streptococci) using the following tests:

1. *Bile solubility*. Pneumococci produce an autolytic enzyme that is capable of lysing the organism's own cell wall during cell growth. When exposed to a bile salt such as sodium deoxycholate, this natural process is accelerated. To perform this test, a drop of 10% sodium deoxycholate is placed on a well-isolated α-hemolytic colony on a blood agar plate. The plate should be left undisturbed for 30 min and when later examined, the colony will have dissolved or flattened if it is a pneumococcus. Other α-hemolytic streptococci are not solubilized by the bile and will be appear unchanged.

2. *Optochin (ethylhydrocupriene hydrochloride) inhibition*. Optochin is capable of lysing pneumococci (positive reaction) but not α-hemolytic streptococci (negative). To perform this test, α-hemolytic colonies are subcultured onto a fresh blood agar plate and an optochin disk is placed in the upper third of the streaked plate. The plate is then incubated overnight at 35°C in 5% CO_2. Organisms that are *S. pneumoniae* will show a zone of inhibition around the disk (Fig. 10.5). α-Hemolytic streptococci will grow up to the edge of the disk.

3. *Latex agglutination test*. This is a rapid slide agglutination procedure that differentiates pneumococci (positive) from α-hemolytic streptococci (negative). To perform the test, a drop of latex reagent is placed onto a black test card. Using a sterile needle or stick, an α-hemolytic colony is removed from a blood agar plate, mixed into the latex reagent, and spread so that the mixture fills the testing area on the card. The card is then rocked back and forth, and the suspension will visibly clump (the background will clear) within 3 min for a positive reaction. The suspension will remain smooth with no clumping for a negative reaction.

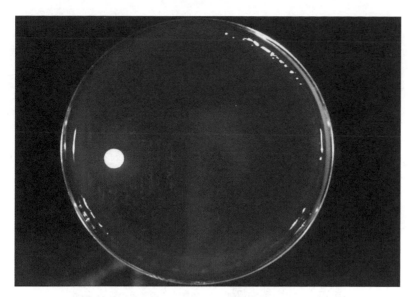

FIGURE 10.5 Blood agar plate with a zone of inhibition surrounding the optochin disk.

The susceptibility of *S. pneumoniae* to antibiotics is tested by determining minimal inhibitory concentrations (MICs) using a microbroth dilution test or by using the E-test method (Fig. 10.6). For a broth microtiter dilution test, serial twofold dilutions of each antimicrobial agent are inoculated with a standardized inoculum of the bacteria and grown overnight in Mueller–Hinton broth. The MIC is read as the lowest concentration of the antibiotic that inhibits the growth of the bacteria. This is the first well where you see no turbidity or growth of the bacteria. For the E-test a range of antibiotic concentrations are placed on a plastic strip, and the bacteria with the strip are incubated for 20–24 h. The MIC for the E-test is read where the zone of inhibition intersects the concentration on the strip. For both methods the MIC (μg/mL) is then interpreted for each antimicrobial agent as susceptible, intermediate, or resistant according to standardized guidelines. Antibiotic susceptibility test results showed our case patient's *S. pneumoniae* isolate to be highly resistant to penicillin (MIC >2 μg/mL), but susceptible to cefotaxime, clindamycin, erythromycin, imipenem, trimethoprim–sulfamethoxazole, levofloxacin, and vancomycin.

10.5. PATHOGENESIS

S. pneumoniae is the most common cause of CAP. In the United States the incidence is 23.2 cases per 100,000, with the majority of cases occurring in the <2- and >65-year-old age groups. One-third of the adult population carries these organisms in their nasopharynx, where it persists as part of their normal flora. *S. pneumoniae* is spread from person to person by aerosols created when someone is coughing, sneezing, or speaking. They can colonize the nasopharynx and invade the body by (1) entering the lungs,

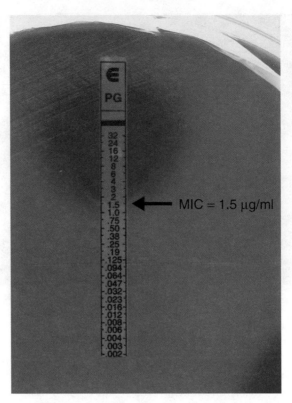

FIGURE 10.6 Antibiotic susceptibility testing by E-test (penicillin) method.

causing pneumonia; (2) entering the eustachian tube, causing ear infection (otitis media); and/or (3) entering the bloodstream, causing sepsis and potentially penetrating further into the meninges, causing meningitis.

Host defenses against pneumococci involve ciliated cells of the upper respiratory tract and the spleen. Cilia are destroyed in people with decreased clearing of the upper airway, such as smokers, and those with chronic asthma, chronic bronchitis, lung cancer, or prior influenza. Without the protective action of the cilia, the pneumococci colonizing the nasopharynx enter the lower respiratory tract, which increases the risk for pneumococcal pneumonia. The spleen acts as a filter to remove bacteria from the blood. Patients who have lost their splenic function due to surgical removal or underlying disease, such as sickle cell disease, are at higher risk for infections with encapsulated bacteria. In addition, patients are also at higher risk for pneumococcal infections if they have chronic diseases, such as systemic lupus erythematosus (SLE), HIV, or multiple myeloma, and if they are taking immunosuppressive drugs or chemotherapeutic agents.

The pneumococcus has many virulence factors, which make it a very effective pathogen. The capsular polysaccharide is a well-known virulence factor that confers antiphagocytic properties to the bacteria and allows them to evade the host macrophages and PMNs. Antibody to the type-specific polysaccharide protects against future infection. However, there are over 90 serotypes of capsular polysaccharide, and antibody to one

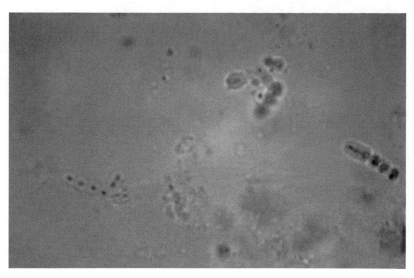

FIGURE 10.7 Positive Quellung reaction.

serotype does not protect against the others. *S. pneumoniae* isolates can be separated into serotypes using antisera directed against the polysaccharide capsule of the organism. A drop of a suspension of the organism is mixed with a drop of specific antiserum plus a drop of methylene blue stain for background color. When specific antisera come in contact with the outer edge of the capsule of the same type, the capsule around the diplococcus appears to plump and swell microscopically. This is called a Quellung reaction (German for "swelling") (Fig. 10.7).

Important virulence factors of *S. pneumoniae* and their mode of action are listed in Table 10.2.

10.6. TREATMENT AND PREVENTION

For the first 30 years that penicillin was available, all *S. pneumoniae* were uniformly susceptible to penicillin at very low concentrations. In 1977 resistance to penicillin developed in South Africa and quickly spread across the world. *S. pneumoniae* acquired two genes that conferred intermediate or high-level resistance to penicillin. The resistance to penicillin is not mediated by β-lactamase production as seen in staphylococci; instead, *S. pneumoniae* can alter their penicillin-binding proteins (PBPs), so that the antibiotic does not bind to the receptor site. Changing the PBPs in bacteria is like changing the lock to a house so that the key (the antibiotic) no longer fits the lock, and therefore does not work.

Our patient has a pneumococcus resistant to penicillin. Alternative antibiotic choices, such as oral macrolides (azithromycin or clarithromycin), effectively treat CAP caused by *S. pneumoniae*, as well as other pathogens causing atypical pneumonia. Ketolide antibiotics (telithromycin) and fluoroquinolones (levofloxacin, ofloxacin) can be used to treat pneumococcal pneumonia since the oral form of these antibiotics has good tissue

TABLE 10.2.	Virulence Factors of *S. pneumoniae* and Their Mode of Action
Virulence Factor	**Characteristics and Activity**
Capsular polysaccharide	Conveys antiphagocytic properties to evade macrophages Evades opsonization of lung surfactant proteins Organisms lacking capsule are avirulent
Adhesion proteins	Allows organisms to bind to disaccharide component of epithelial cells Used instead of pili or fimbriae to adhere to human cells
Secretory IgA protease	Helps bacteria avoid entrapment in mucus
Pneumolysin	A cytotoxin released when bacteria lyse Allows organism to bypass clearance mechanisms of upper airway Destroys ciliated cells Binds to cholesterol in host cell membrane and disrupts cells by forming pores (action similar to that of streptolysin O) Decreases the oxidative burst of monocytes and PMNs
Hydrogen peroxide	Causes tissue damage Provides bacteria with nutrients Protects bacteria from phagocytes in damaged areas
Choline	Part of the pneumococcal cell wall Enables bacterial cell to bind to platelet activating factor (PAF) receptors and enter the host cell in an endocytic vacuole Facilitates invasion into alveolar cells
Peptidoglycan and teichoic acid	Cell wall components with activity analogous to lipopolysaccharide in gram-negative bacteria Activates alternative complement pathway Induces production of cytokines (IL-1 and TNF-α and PAF)

penetration. However, resistance has been documented to all these antibiotics, and susceptibility testing may be required to select an appropriate antimicrobial agent.

Pneumonia caused by pneumococci that have intermediate resistance to penicillin can be treated with higher doses of penicillin, but when the penicillin MIC is ≥ 2 μg/mL, the antibiotic should be avoided. Third-generation cephalosporins (ceftriaxone, cefotaxime) can be used to treat serious pneumococcal infections. The MIC to ceftriaxone or cefotaxime is interpreted differently for meningitis and nonmeningitis infections since the concentration of these antibiotics is lower in the cerebrospinal fluid (CSF) compared to levels in the blood, lungs or sinuses. The recommended therapy for patients with pneumococcal meningitis is to combine either ceftriaxone or cefotaxime with vancomycin until susceptibility results are known. Vancomycin can be discontinued if the organisms are susceptible to the β-lactam antibiotics.

To prevent serious pneumococcal disease in both adults and children, vaccines are available that contain multiple polysaccharide antigens. An adult vaccine containing 23 purified capsular polysaccharide antigens is recommended for the elderly and for those with underlying cardiac and lung diseases. The 23 serotypes chosen for the vaccine represent 85–90% of the serotypes that cause invasive disease in the United States. Children under 2 do not respond to the 23-valent vaccine since polysaccharide antigens are less immunogenic than proteins. A pediatric vaccine (Prevnar) was recently developed that couples nine polysaccharide antigens to a nonpneumococcal protein, making it immunogenic in children as young as two months of age. The pneumococcal conjugate vaccine has been added to the recommended vaccines for children younger than 2 years of age in the United States by the Advisory Committee on Immunization Practices of the Centers for Disease Control and Prevention and the American Academy of Pediatrics.

10.7. ADDITIONAL POINTS

■ A microbiologic diagnosis is obtained in only 50–70% of patients with community acquired pneumonia. Of patients with pneumococcal pneumonia, 20–30% will have a positive blood culture, and yet half of patients with positive blood cultures will have negative sputum cultures. Hence, blood culture may be the only way to make a diagnosis for some patients.

■ The preferred tests for the diagnosis of *Legionella pneumophila* are a urinary antigen assay, and culture using selective media. While results are available more rapidly with the urinary antigen test compared to culture, a disadvantage of the test is that it detects antigen of only *L. pneumophila* serogroup 1. The sensitivity of this test is 80% with a high specificity (>95%). Culture detects all 14 serogroups of *L. pneumophila* as well as other *Legionella* species. Colonies can appear in 3–4 days; however, cultures are held for as long as 2 weeks before discarding. A direct fluorescent antibody test performed on respiratory specimens is available for *Legionella* testing; however, it suffers from poor sensitivity (25–75%). Because it is highly specific (95%), the test is helpful if positive. Because sputum from patients with *Legionella* is frequently nonpurulent and watery, the screening system used to evaluate the quality of sputum is not applicable. Respiratory specimens should be transported without holding media or saline, which can inhibit the growth of *Legionella* spp.

■ Identification of *Haemophilus influenzae* as the etiologic agent of CAP is achieved by sputum culture. In children, *H. influenzae* can also cause sinusitis, otitis, and epiglottitis. On Gram stain the organism is a "pleomorphic" gram-negative rod, meaning that it appears to be coccobacillary. All *Haemophilus* species require accessory X (hemin) and/or V [nicotine adenine dinucleotide (NAD)] factors for growth (Fig. 10.8). They do not grow on 5% blood sheep blood agar or MacConkey agar. Chocolate

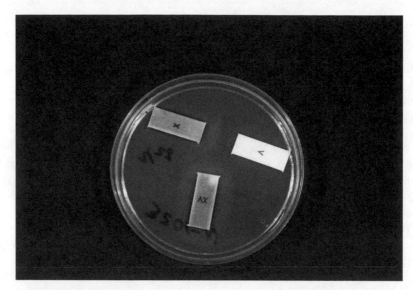

FIGURE 10.8 Growth of *Haemophilus influenzae* around X and V factors.

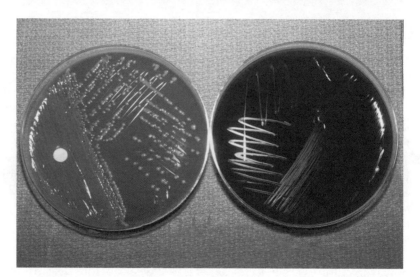

FIGURE 10.9 Colonies of *Haemophilus influenzae* on chocolate agar (left) and no growth on blood agar (right).

agar containing X and V factors will support the growth of *Haemophilus* when the agar is incubated at 35°C in an atmosphere of 5–8% CO_2 (Fig. 10.9). Growth of *Haemophilus* can been as satelliting colonies around *S. aureus*, which hemolyzes the RBCs providing the necessary X and V factors (Fig. 10.10). *Haemophilus* are classified into species on the basis of their X- and V-factor requirements and β-hemolysis on horse blood (Table 10.3). *H. influenzae* can be further subdivided into typable and nontypable strains according to the presence or absence of a polyribitol phosphate capsule. *H. influenzae* encapsulated strains are divided into six groups: types a, b, c, d, e, and f. Pneumonia and serious systemic

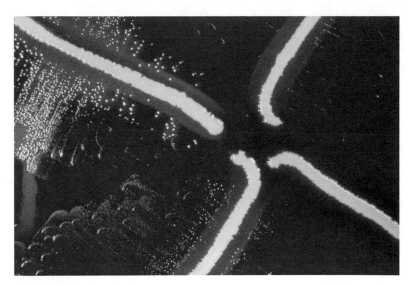

FIGURE 10.10 Satellite colonies of *Haemophilus influenzae* around *Staphylococcus aureus.*

TABLE 10.3.	Growth Factors Required by *Haemophilus* Species			
	Growth on Agar Containing			
Organism	X Factor	V Factor	X and V Factors	Hemolysis
H. aphrophilus	+	−	+	−
H. ducreyi	+	−	+	−
H. influenzae	−	−	+	−
H. parainfluenzae	−	+	ı	−
H. hemolyticus	−	−	+	+
H. parahemolyticus	−	+	+	+

disease is most commonly caused by encapsulated strains; nontypable *H. influenzae* are normal upper respiratory flora. Prior to introduction of the vaccine in 1990, *H. influenzae* type b (Hib) was a major cause of meningitis, septicemia, epiglottitis, and serious systemic illness in children. Widespread use and acceptance of the vaccine has made this a rare occurrence.

■ In children, the common causes of CAP in normal hosts include *S. pneumoniae*, *S. aureus*, *H. influenzae*, *M. tuberculosis*, *M. pneumoniae*, *C. pneumoniae*, and *C. trachomatis*; respiratory syncytial virus; influenza A or B; parainfluenza viruses 1, 2, and 3; adenovirus; rhinovirus; and measles virus.

■ Serologic tests are available for the diagnosis of *Mycoplasma pneumoniae*, *Chlamydia pneumoniae*, and other less frequently seen pathogens that should not be screened for routinely. If suspected, serum should be frozen and saved for future testing.

SUGGESTED READING

FILE, T. M., Clinical implications and treatment of multiresistant *Streptococcus pneumoniae* pneumonia, *Clin. Microbiol. Infect.* **12** (Suppl. 3):31–41 (2006).

MANDELL, L. A., Antimicrobial resistance and treatment of community-acquired pneumonia, *Clin. Chest Med.* **26**:57–64 (2005).

MANDELL L. A., R. G. WUNDERINK, A. ANZUETO, J. G. BARTLETT, G. D. CAMPBELL, N. C. DEAN, S. F. DOWELL, T. M. FILE, JR., D. M. MUSHER, M. S. NIEDERMAN, A. TORRES, AND C. G. WHITNEY, Infectious Diseases Society of America/American Thoracic Society Consensus Guidelines on the Management of Community-Acquired Pneumonia in Adults, *Clin. Infect. Dis.* **44** (Suppl 2):S27–S72 (2007).

MCINTOSH, K., Community-acquired pneumonia in children, *N. Engl. J. Med.* **346**:429–37 (2002).

ORTQVIST, A., J. HEDLUND, AND M. KALIN, *Streptococcus pneumoniae*: Epidemiology, risk factors, and clinical features, *Semin. Resp. Crit. Care Med.* **26**:563–574 (2005).

Nursing Home Resident with Fever, Cough, and Myalgias

11.1. PATIENT HISTORY

The patient is an 82 year-old female nursing home resident who is brought to the emergency department in late December with the chief complaint of abrupt onset of fever, chills, and nonproductive cough. She also complains of severe muscle aches (myalgias) and headaches. The patient mentioned that she had seen many visitors over the holidays, particularly her grandchildren, some of whom were complaining of muscle aches and fever. Of note, she has not received any vaccinations within the last 3 years. She has no chronic diseases and does not smoke.

On physical exam (PE) the patient was ill-appearing, but did not appear toxic. Her temperature was 39.4°C (103°F), her throat was red (erythematous), but no exudates were noted, and she had a clear nasal discharge. There was no lymphadenopathy. Her lungs were clear. The remainder of her PE was unremarkable. A chest x-ray was within normal limits.

11.2. DIFFERENTIAL DIAGNOSIS

While this patient presents with symptoms suggesting multisystem disease, the major system involved appears to be the upper respiratory tract. Epidemiologic factors to note in this case include the season of the year, the patient's age, the patient's residence, and recent contact with multiple

Medical Microbiology for the New Curriculum: A Case-Based Approach, by Roberta B. Carey, Mindy G. Schuster, and Karin L. McGowan.
Copyright © 2008 John Wiley & Sons, Inc.

family members exposing the patient to agents prevalent in the community. Likely diagnoses include viral or bacterial upper respiratory infection, *Streptococcus pneumoniae* pneumonia, and atypical pneumonia. The latter two options become much less likely in this patient because of her negative chest x-ray. When influenza virus is prevalent in the community, most persons from the community presenting with an acute febrile respiratory illness and negative chest x-ray should be assumed to have an influenza virus infection. In addition, the fact that this nursing home resident has not been immunized against influenza places her at even greater risk. Age > 60 years is a major risk factor for developing complications from influenza.

Infectious Causes

Bacteria

Legionella spp.

Mycoplasma pneumoniae

Streptococcus pneumoniae

Streptococcus pyogenes (group A streptococci)

Fungi

Fungi are an unlikely cause of upper respiratory infection in a normal host.

Parasites

Parasites are an unlikely cause of upper respiratory infection.

Viruses

Adenovirus

Corona virus [severe acute respiratory syndrome (SARS)]

Influenza A and B viruses

Parainfluenza virus

Respiratory syncytial virus (RSV)

Rhinoviruses

CLINICAL CLUES

? Abnormal breath sounds (consolidation) on pulmonary exam? For patients with bacterial pneumonia, changes are usually noted on physical exam; for patients with influenza, the exam is usually unremarkable.

? Continued fever and progression of shortness of breath for more than 4–5 days? Suspect influenza pneumonia, a severe complication of influenza.

? Symptoms initially improve, and then worsen 2–3 days later? Suspect a secondary bacterial pneumonia.

11.3. LABORATORY TESTS

While the diagnosis of influenza is frequently based on signs and symptoms, laboratory diagnosis and confirmation is highly recommended because the symptoms of influenza are not easily distinguishable from those caused by other respiratory pathogens. The laboratory diagnosis of influenza A and B viruses can be made by direct staining of respiratory tract secretions using fluorescent antibody (FA), membrane enzyme immunoassay (EIA) tests, conventional cell culture, shell vial culture, and serologic testing. Membrane EIA tests are very rapid (<1 h), have a sensitivity range of 70–90%, and are used by many hospitals for rapid testing during winter viral season. Some detect only influenza A viruses, others detect both influenza A and B viruses. Because EIA tests are less sensitive than culture, specimens yielding negative EIA test results should be further tested by FA staining or culture. FA staining involves the direct detection of virus-infected cells using monoclonal antibody reagents and immunofluorescent microscopy. It can be used to detect RSV, influenza, parainfluenza, and adenovirus on the same slide. In terms of sensitivity and specificity, FA staining is considered equivalent to culture for influenzas A and B.

Viral culture involves inoculation of specimens into cell cultures, incubation of cell cultures, observation of cell cultures for characteristic cytopathic effect (CPE), and finally further identification by method, such as hemadsorption and fluorescent monoclonal antibodies specific for influenza virus A or B. Influenza virus is easily grown in cell culture, and positive cultures can be obtained within 4 days. The shell vial technique for rapid (within 24 h) detection of viruses can be also be used to detect influenza A and B viruses. Submitting specimens for viral culture is important because only culture isolates when submitted to state and reference laboratories can supply valuable information on the influenza subtypes and strains circulating in the community. Viral isolates also help in monitoring the emergence of antiviral resistance in the community.

Influenza-specific antibodies can be detected as soon as 4–7 days after the onset of symptoms following a primary infection with influenza and reach peak levels 3–4 weeks after onset of symptoms. Antibody tests should not be used to diagnose acute disease because paired sera (acute and convalescent sera taken 10–14 days apart) must be tested and then examined for a fourfold rise in titer for a diagnosis.

For best results, specimens should be collected within 3 days of the onset of illness. Nasopharyngeal (NP) washings, bronchoalveolar lavage specimens, and NP swabs are the specimens of choice for diagnosing influenza. Once collected, specimens should be placed in a viral transport medium. Specimens for viral isolation should not be allowed to sit at room temperature. They should be placed on ice (not frozen) and transported immediately or refrigerated until transport is possible.

Because this patient was well-appearing and had a negative chest x-ray, a nasal aspirate was taken and submitted for influenza EIA testing and complete viral culture. Two pretreatment sets of blood cultures, as well as a Gram stain and culture of pretreatment expectorated sputum, were also submitted for routine bacterial culture.

11.4. RESULTS

The nasal aspirate specimen submitted for rapid testing was positive for influenza by EIA (Fig. 11.1). Viral culture performed on the same specimen and stained with fluorescent-labeled antibody to influenza A virus was positive (Fig. 11.2), and the isolate was forwarded to the state public health department, where it was further identified. Nomenclature of influenza viruses is based on the virus type, the geographic location where the virus was first isolated, a laboratory identification number, and the year of

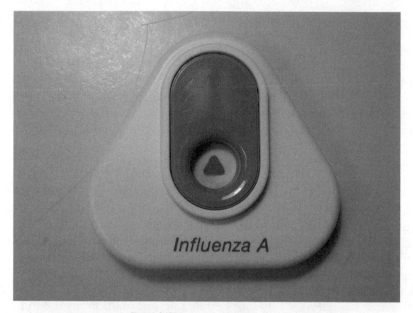

FIGURE 11.1 Rapid EIA test (positive) for influenza A.

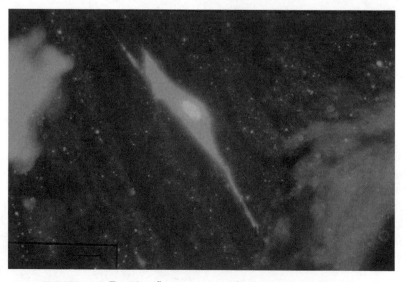

FIGURE 11.2 Positive fluorescent antibody test for influenza.

isolation followed by the subtype. Our patient's isolate was characterized as influenza A/Panama/2007/99 (H3N2). Both rapid streptococcal antigen testing and culture were negative for group A streptococcus. The Gram stain of the patient's sputum specimen was considered inadequate for culture (predominance of squamous epithelial cells with few WBCs), and no further bacteriology was performed.

11.5. PATHOGENESIS

Influenza belongs to the family of orthomyxoviruses, which are enveloped viruses with segmented RNA. There are three major antigenic types; influenza A, B, and C. Influenza B circulates only among humans, but influenza A is found in humans and many different animals, including ducks, pigs, chickens, and horses. The eight RNA segments of influenza A can be recombined with the RNA segments from influenza found in animals and create a completely new strain of virus. When the influenza A virus undergoes a major reassortment of antigens into a new viral strain, this is known as "antigenic shift," and it may lead to a pandemic since no one has previous immunity to the virus. "Antigenic drift" occurs when minor changes occur in the genome as a result of mutations, which results in the annual seasonal epidemic. In the Northern Hemisphere, influenza season usually begins in November and lasts until April. However, the timing of influenza activity varies from year to year. It is not necessary to test for influenza infection until the winter season unless the patient has a travel history to Alaska or the Far East, where the virus circulates earlier. Influenza C is a milder respiratory illness and does not result in epidemics.

On the surface of the influenza virus there are two major glycoproteins; the hemagglutinin (HA) and neuraminidase (NA) (Fig. 11.3). HA and NA are the key antigens for the virus that can be reshuffled into different antigenic types. HA is responsible for viral attachment. It binds to the sialic acid moiety on the host epithelial cell and facilitates fusion of the host and viral membranes. To date 16 antigenic types of hemagglutinin (H1, H2, H3,... H16) and nine neuraminidase types (N1, N2, N3,..., N9) have been reported. NA cleaves the sialic acid residues and allows the newly formed

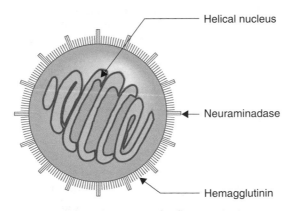

Helical nucleus

Neuraminadase

Hemagglutinin

FIGURE 11.3 Structure of influenza A virus.

virions to be released from the host cell. Two types of NA are commonly found in human influenza A infections (N1 and N2). Antibodies raised to the HA and NA are protective and type-specific; therefore the antibodies will not prevent future infection if the HA and NA antigens change.

Although influenza causes a significant amount of illness and loss of time at work and school, it is usually self-limiting, and most people recover in 5–7 days. High-risk patients can develop complications or die. The only organ that influenza infects is the lung, but the symptoms of influenza are systemic. The virus is spread from person to person by respiratory droplets from sneezing, coughing, kissing, and contact with respiratory secretions on beverage glasses and other objects (fomites). Adults may be contagious from one day before symptoms start up to seven days after getting sick. Children may shed the virus for longer periods of time. The influenza virus stimulates an inflammatory cell response of lymphocytes and monoctyes in the upper respiratory tract. The virus binds to host cells, enters cell cytoplasm, uncoats to expose its RNA, multiplies (replicates), and causes cell death. The infection is stopped when sufficient cell-mediated immunity and interferon are produced.

An estimated 10–20% of U.S. residents get the flu annually. On average, 114,000 persons are hospitalized for flu-related complications, and 36,000 Americans die each year from complications of influenza. The most common complication is pneumonia. Those at the extremes of age (young children and the elderly) are at the highest risk for infection. The majority of deaths seen during annual influenza epidemics occur in patients greater than 65 years of age, especially those in chronic care facilities. Pregnant women are also at risk since their cellular immunity is depressed during the third trimester to prevent rejection of the fetus. Patients with underlying cardiac and lung disease have a more severe illness and may have significant complications. It is possible for influenza to rapidly proceed to pneumonia and to progress into acute respiratory distress syndrome (ARDS). This is more likely to occur in patients with cardiovascular or chronic pulmonary disease or in pregnant women. Infection of the heart muscles (myocarditis) and pericardium (pericarditis) are rare complications that have also been associated with influenza.

Secondary bacterial pneumonia is the most important complication associated with influenza and should be anticipated when managing elderly patients. Secondary bacterial infection may begin 5–7 days after the onset of viral symptoms and is associated with a rapid worsening of clinical symptoms after the initial illness has begun to resolve. The initial viral infection depletes the cilia on the tracheobronchial epithelial cells, which allows bacteria to penetrate deeper into the respiratory tract. *S. pneumoniae* is the most common cause of secondary bacterial pneumonia, but pneumonia due to *Staphylococcus aureus* and *Haemophilus influenzae* can occur as well.

11.6. TREATMENT AND PREVENTION

If the diagnosis is made within 48 h of infection, antiviral agents may be given to ameliorate the symptoms and decrease the length of time that the virus is shed. Oral amantadine or rimantadine inhibit the uncoating of influenza A, but are ineffective against influenza B. Amantadine is excreted unchanged in the urine and is associated with CNS side effects. Rimantadine is metabolized in the liver, and a lower dose is recommended for patients with liver disease, renal failure, and elderly nursing home residents. Newer antivirals, zanamivir, an inhaled compound, and oseltamivir, an oral compound, inhibit both influenza A and B viruses by restricting viral NA activity. Amantadine, rimantadine, and oseltamivir have been FDA-approved for chemoprophylaxis to prevent infection in those at highest risk after exposure.

Annual vaccination is the best method of preventing infection. Because different strains of influenza virus circulate each year, a new vaccine is formulated to induce immunity to the latest antigenic variant. The U.S. vaccines are formalin-inactivated viruses that are disrupted with detergents (split-product vaccines). The virus is grown in chick eggs, and those with severe allergic reactions to egg protein should not receive the vaccine.

Annual vaccination is recommended for those over 65 years of age, those with chronic diseases (heart, lung, kidney disease, HIV or other immunosuppressive conditions), women who will be in the second or third trimester of pregnancy during flu season, and healthcare workers. It is very important that healthcare workers be protected from infection to avoid transmitting the virus to patients who are under their care. The vaccine is encouraged for children 6–23 months of age and their caregivers either at home or in daycare. A new vaccine administered intranasally of a live, cold-adapted influenza virus was approved in 2003 to immunize healthy individuals 5–50 years of age.

11.7. ADDITIONAL POINTS

■ Intramuscularly administered influenza vaccine is a killed virus vaccine and cannot cause influenza. The most common side effect associated with the vaccine is soreness at the injection site.

■ Reye's syndrome is an extrapulmonary complication of influenza B and can also follow infection with influenza A and varicella. This complication is associated with influenza in children and teenagers and carries a fatality rate of 10%. This syndrome develops 2–12 days after onset of infection and is characterized by cerebral edema and severe fatty infiltration of the liver. It is thought to be associated with aspirin and other salicylate ingestion. There has been a marked reduction in the incidence of Reye's syndrome since warnings have been issued against aspirin treatment for viral illness.

■ Infection with parainfluenza virus may mimic influenza infections, although the symptoms are not as severe. Parainfluenza viruses circulate in the fall and spring seasons and are associated with outbreaks of croup. Immunocomprised patients may develop a more prolonged respiratory illness with parainfluenza virus infection. Antivirals against influenza are not effective against the parainfluenza viruses.

■ The introduction of new viral infections such as severe acute respiratory syndrome (SARS) may make the differential diagnosis of influenza challenging, and in this setting, laboratory confirmation may be essential.

SARS should be suspected in individuals with symptoms consistent with influenza who have been exposed to a person with SARS or have traveled to an area with active cases within 10 days.

■ *Mycobacterium tuberculosis* should always be considered when evaluating nursing home residents with pneumonia and a positive chest x-ray. Nursing home residents account for 20% of tuberculosis cases seen in the elderly, and the incidence of active tuberculosis is 10–30 times greater among nursing home residents compared to elderly adults living in the community. Tuberculosis usually causes more chronic symptoms.

SUGGESTED READING

CDC, Prevention and control of influenza: Recommendations of the advisory committee on immunization practices (ACIP), *MMWR* **55**(RR-10):1–42 (2006).

EBELL, M. H., Diagnosing and treating patients with suspected influenza, *Am. Fam. Physician* **72**:1789–1792 (2005).

FALSEY, A. R. AND E. E. WALSH, Viral pneumonia in older adults, *Clin. Infect. Dis.* **42**:518–524 (2006).

RUIZ, M., S. EWIG, M. A. MARCOS, J. A. MARTINEZ, F. ARANCIBIA, J. MENSA, AND A. TORRES, Etiology of community-acquired pneumonia: Impact of age, co-morbidity, and severity, *Am. J. Crit. Care Med.* **160**:397–405 (1999).

www.cdc.gov/flu.

Baby with Fever, Rhinitis and Bronchiolitis

12.1. PATIENT HISTORY

The patient is a 6 month-old healthy infant boy brought to the hospital emergency department (ED) in early December with a three-day history of low-grade fever, runny nose (rhinitis), and a nonproductive cough. On physical exam (PE), he was slightly agitated and coughing but in mild respiratory distress. His vital signs were temperature 37.8°C (100°F), heart rate 140 beats/min, blood pressure 90/70 mm Hg, and a respiratory rate of 60–80 breaths/min with grunting and retractions. The remainder of the PE was normal. Of note, he has been attending daycare for the past two months, and his one sibling (2 years of age) was reported to be coughing at home as well. His immunizations are up-to-date.

A chest x-ray was obtained and showed marked increased lung volumes, with evidence of hyperaeration. Moderate peribronchial cuffing due to bronchial wall thickening and edema was also noted. No pleural fluid (effusion) was present, and radiology commented that the chest x-ray findings were consistent with viral bronchiolitis. Laboratory findings were as follows: WBC count, 8100/mm^3 and normal blood electrolytes. Arterial blood gas revealed normal oxygenation, with a mild respiratory alkalosis. Because of the patient's nasal discharge and cough, nasopharyngeal washings were obtained in the ED and sent to the laboratory for rapid respiratory syncytial virus (RSV) and influenza testing. Laboratory data were notable for a positive RSV test and a negative influenza types A and B

Medical Microbiology for the New Curriculum: A Case-Based Approach, by Roberta B. Carey, Mindy G. Schuster, and Karin L. McGowan.
Copyright © 2008 John Wiley & Sons, Inc.

test. After the physician instructed the parents, the patient was discharged to home.

12.2. DIFFERENTIAL DIAGNOSIS

Bronchiolitis is the term used for inflammation of the small air passages in the lungs called bronchioles, and it is usually viral in nature. Bronchiolitis is usually seen in infants less than 2 years of age, and the highest incidence occurs in infants less than 6 months old. It is most common in winter and early spring in temperate climates. A more severe illness may be experienced by patients with congenital heart disease, cystic fibrosis, chronic lung disease, organ and bone marrow transplantation, and immunodeficiencies. Causes of bronchiolitis include those listed below.

Infectious Causes

Bacteria

> *Bordetella pertussis*
>
> *Mycoplasma pneumoniae*

Viruses

> Adenovirus
>
> Human metapneumovirus
>
> Influenza virus (both A and B)
>
> Measles (measles bronchiolitis is incredibly rare in the United States and other countries where most people have been vaccinated)
>
> Parainfluenza virus types 1, 2, and 3
>
> Respiratory syncytial virus (RSV)
>
> Rhinovirus

Fungi

> Fungi are not a cause of bronchiolitis.

Parasites

> Parasites are not a cause of bronchiolitis.

Noninfectious Causes

> Airway hypersensitivity
>
> Asthma
>
> Gastroesophageal reflux with aspiration

CLINICAL CLUES

? Fever, cough, coryza, and rhinorrhea in a child less than two years of age in the winter? Think RSV, which can also be associated with otitis media and conjunctivitis.

? Wheezing on expiration in a child less than two years of age in the winter? Think RSV.

? A noninfluenza respiratory illness in an elderly resident of a nursing home? Think RSV. Patients with influenza often have more impressive myalgias.

? An infant with upper respiratory symptoms and apnea? Think of RSV. In up to 20% of infants admitted to the hospital with RSV, apnea will be the presenting symptom, and premature infants are at highest risk.

12.3. LABORATORY TESTS

Blood cultures and nasopharyngeal aspirate specimens were obtained and sent to the microbiology laboratory. Rapid testing plus culture for respiratory viruses and polymerase chain reaction (PCR) for *Bordetella pertussis* were requested. There are several ways to test for respiratory viruses. Conventional cell culture, shell vial culture, rapid antigen detection by direct immunofluorescent assay (DFA) or enzyme immunoassay (EIA) for RSV and influenzae types A and B, and molecular methods (e.g., real-time PCR) are all excellent ways to make the laboratory diagnosis.

Respiratory viruses grow in a variety of different cell lines. Conventional tube (Fig. 12.1) cultures take 5–8 days postinoculation to produce

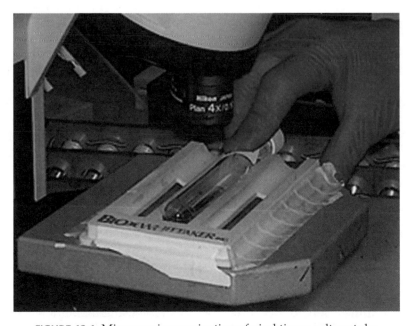

FIGURE 12.1 Microscopic examination of viral tissue culture tube.

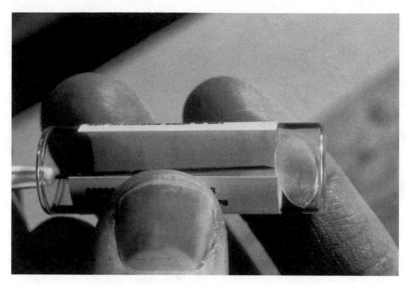

FIGURE 12.2 Shell vial tube with coverslip.

cytopathic effect (CPE). The shell vial technique is used to shorten the time required to detect viruses in culture. A vial containing a monolayer of a cell line growing on a circular coverslip is inoculated with the specimen, and then the vial is centrifuged to speed the attachment and incorporation of virus into the cell line (Fig. 12.2). A shell vial containing a mix of different cell lines can grow a variety of respiratory viruses in a single vial. Isolated viruses are then identified using techniques such as fluorescent antibody staining, neutralization assays, or adherence of red blood cells onto the infected cells (hemadsorption). While sensitive and specific, isolation of respiratory viruses by cell culture is not rapid enough to influence patient management.

Antigen detection methods (DFA and EIA) are rapid when compared to culture and can identify a virus directly from a clinical specimen in a few hours. For viruses such as influenza and RSV, obtaining results in hours rather than days allows for better control of nosocomial infections and allows newly admitted patients to be cohorted appropriately. For infections where antiviral therapy is an option, it also allows for more appropriate use of antivirals and avoids the inappropriate use of antibiotics. Immunofluorescence (DFA) assays simultaneously test for antigens of RSV, influenza virus types A and B, adenovirus, and parainfluenza virus types 1, 2, and 3. DFA staining detects viral antigens that are expressed in respiratory epithelial cells (Fig. 12.3). The critical aspect of DFA testing is the quality of the specimen submitted to the lab because specimens must contain an adequate number of respiratory epithelial cells. Most labs require 50–100 cells to consider a specimen adequate. The best specimens are nasopharyngeal or tracheal aspirates, nasal washes, bronchoalveolar fluid, or nasopharyngeal swabs. EIA tests detect cell-free antigens as well as antigen in epithelial cells. They can be adapted for automated instruments for large volume testing or performed one at a time using membrane test devices (Figs. 12.4, 12.5). EIA methods have become even more popular than

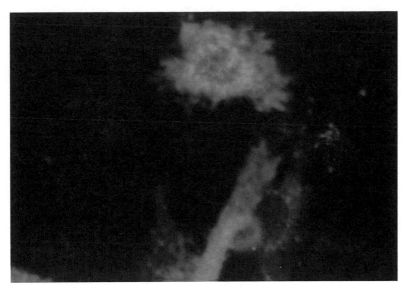

FIGURE 12.3 Direct fluorescent antibody staining of RSV-infected cell.

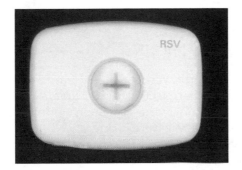

FIGURE 12.4 Positive rapid EIA test for RSV.

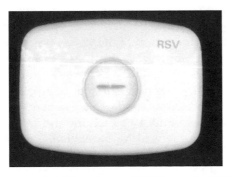

FIGURE 12.5 Negative rapid EIA test for RSV.

DFA because they can be performed by less technically trained personnel and do not require a fluorescent microscope. Both membrane–enzyme immunoassay and DFA have sensitivity approaching culture. While a positive rapid test is critical for management decisions involving treatment and infection control, all negatives should be followed up with culture.

While not widely available at this time, real-time PCR (RT-PCR) is being used for the detection of respiratory viruses. When used to simultaneously test a panel of respiratory viruses (multiplex), it provides a rapid and accurate method for detection of coinfections with multiple viruses in a single assay. At the moment, the cost of RT-PCR is prohibitive for wide-scale use. For most hospitals, the use of rapid fluorescence and EIA methods with cell culture to confirm negatives is less expensive and meets clinical needs.

12.4. RESULTS

The nasopharyngeal aspirate specimen was positive for RSV and negative for influenza types A and B using a rapid EIA assay. Viral culture revealed no additional pathogens. Blood cultures for bacterial pathogens were negative. PCR for *B. pertussis* was negative.

12.5. PATHOGENESIS

RSV is a major cause of lower respiratory infection among young children resulting in more than 50,000 hospitalizations annually in the United States, where it is a seasonal virus causing major outbreaks from November to March each year. Premature infants and children with chronic lung disease or with hemodynamically significant heart disease are more likely to have increased morbidity and mortality with RSV infections. RSV also causes severe illness in adults over 65 years of age, and in persons with underlying respiratory or cardiac disease or compromised immune systems. Chronic obstructive pulmonary disease (COPD), coronary vascular disease, and smoking are known risk factors for more severe disease in older adults.

RSV is a paramyxovirus related to parainfluenza, measles, mumps, and metapneumovirus in the genus *Pneumovirus*. The name respiratory syncytial virus reflects the action of the virus on infected cells that clump together, loosing their unique cell wall and forming one giant cell, or syncytia (Fig. 12.6). It is an enveloped single-stranded RNA virus, whose viability is subject to temperature extremes. Unlike influenza, RSV lacks the virulence factors of neuraminadase and hemagglutinin proteins. RSV directly invades the respiratory epithelium and stimulates lymphocytic infiltrate with edema in the walls of bronchioles and surrounding tissue. Immunologically mediated injury causes necrosis of the epithelium leading to obstruction of the small airways from the sloughed epithelial cells and increased mucus. Inflow and outflow of air is impeded, and air is

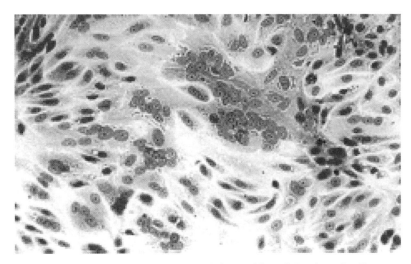

FIGURE 12.6 Giant cell (syncytia) formed by RSV-infected cells.

trapped in the lungs, causing hyperinflation and wheezing. Trapped air is absorbed and results in incomplete expansion of the lung (atelectasis).

RSV may mimic the common cold, or cause a more serious illness of bronchiolitis or pneumonia. It does not have a viremic phase, and a secondary bacterial infection is very rare in RSV patients. However, a 1–3% case fatality rate is seen in premature infants in intensive care nurseries.

12.6. TREATMENT AND PREVENTION

Treatment for RSV infection is primarily supportive. Oxygen administration, IV fluids, and nebulized cold steam are used to ameliorate the symptoms. If wheezing is present, a trial of bronchodilators can be considered. Antiviral medication is not used routinely unless the patient has severe underlying disease. Inhaled ribavirin, a synthetic nucleoside, has activity against RSV, but it is associated with risks for the healthcare worker, is expensive, and is of unclear benefit, and thus, not routinely recommended. Our patient was considered a normal host, who did not require hospitalization. He was released to his parents' care, and they were advised to bring him back if he showed signs of worsening, such as increased respiratory rate, labored breathing, or signs of dehydration.

RSV is highly contagious and is considered an important nosocomial pathogen. The incubation period lasts 4–5 days, and infected patients can shed high quantities of the virus for weeks. The virus can be carried by healthcare workers and visitors, and the virus can survive on fomites, such as countertops, for more than 24 h or spread in large droplets from the secretions of an infected person. Strict adherence to infection control practices, especially good hand hygiene, is required to prevent transmission. New admissions suspected of having RSV, or those with a positive rapid diagnostic test for RSV, are isolated or cohorted with other RSV infected patients.

IgM, IgG, and IgA are produced in response to the RSV infection, but natural immunity does not protect against reinfection, although the second time the virus is encountered the disease is less severe. Passive immunotherapy with RSV immunoglobulin has not been proved effective for treatment of infection. Infection can be prevented with palivizumab, a humanized monoclonal antibody produced to the fusion protein on the surface of the virus (F protein). Immunoprophylaxis may be given to premature infants and children with congenital heart disease, who are at the highest risk for increased morbidity and mortality from the disease. The financial cost for this program in a neonatal nursery is significant since the antibody must be administered monthly throughout the RSV season to be protective.

No vaccine is currently available. Early studies with a whole-cell viral vaccine showed more severe disease in the vaccine recipients, but trials are underway with an attenuated subunit vaccine that shows promise.

12.7. ADDITIONAL POINTS

■ There are several indications for hospitalization in bronchiolitis caused by RSV:

1. Age < 3 months

2. Hypoxemia and need for oxygen

3. Underlying cardiopulmonary disease or immunodeficiencies

4. Atelectasis or consolidation on chest radiography

5. Wheezing and respiratory distress associated with oxygen saturation below 92%

6. Dehydration and poor oral intake

■ In 2001, the human metapneumovirus was identified as a new respiratory virus. It has been isolated from nasopharyngeal aspirates of both children and adults with acute respiratory tract infections. The infections range from a mild respiratory illness to severe bronchiolitis and pneumonia. While the importance of this virus is still unknown, serology studies have shown that by age 5 years, almost all children have been in contact with the virus. Initial studies have revealed that this virus may be an important pathogen in young children (<3 years) and the elderly.

■ The laboratory diagnosis of *B. pertussis* can be made by direct fluorescent antibody (DFA) testing of nasopharyngeal swab or aspirate, culture, PCR, or serology. PCR is considered the most sensitive assay and is not affected by phase of the disease (early, catarrhal, paroxysmal) or prior antibiotic use. Culture is considered no more than 50% sensitive because of issues related to specimen collection and transport, the fastidious nature of the organism, and interference from other bacterial flora. Reagents for DFA testing have variable sensitivity and low specificity, and as a result, a positive DFA result without culture or PCR confirmation is not considered suitable confirmation of pertussis.

SUGGESTED READING

BONNET, D., A. A. SCHMALTZ, AND T. F. FELTES, Infection by the respiratory syncytial virus in infants and young children at high risk, *Cardiol. Young.* **15**:256–265 (2005).

CDC, Pertussis—United States, 2001–2003, *MMWR* **54**:1283–1286 (2005).

CHIDGEY, S. M. AND K. J. BROADLEY, Respiratory syncytial virus infections: Characteristics and treatment, *J. Pharm. Pharmacol.* **57**:1371–1381 (2005).

FALSEY, A. R., P. A. HENNESSEY, M. A. FORMICA, C. COX, AND E. E. WALSH, Respiratory syncytial virus infection in elderly and high risk adults, *N. Engl. J. Med.* **352**:1749–1759 (2005).

LEIDY, N. K., M. K. MARGOLIS, J. P. MARCIN, J. A. FLYNN, L. R. FRANKEL, S. JOHNSON, D. LANGKAMP, AND E. A. SIMOES, The impact of severe respiratory syncytial virus on the child, caregiver, and family during hospitalization and recovery. *Pediatrics*, **115**:1536–1546 (2005).

Woman with Fever, Cough, and Weight Loss

13.1. PATIENT HISTORY

A 56 year-old Vietnamese woman presents with fever, cough, and a 10 lb weight loss over the preceding 2 months. Her cough is productive of whitish sputum that is occasionally tinged with blood. She also reports night sweats for the past 3 weeks. She was born in Vietnam and came to the United States 20 years ago. She has not returned since and has had no other significant travel. She reports having had a Bacillus Calmette-Guérin (BCG) vaccine as a child. She recalls that her grandmother, who had lived with her, was ill with a "bad pneumonia" for several months when she was a young child. She lives with her husband and two teenage children, who are all in good health. She denies use of alcohol, tobacco, or intravenous drugs or any risk factors for human immunodeficiency virus (HIV).

Physical examination reveals a very thin woman in no acute distress. Her temperature is 38.5°C (101.3°F), heart rate 90 beats/min, blood pressure 100/68 mm Hg, and respiratory rate 18 breaths/min. She is breathing comfortably. There are no skin or oral lesions. There is no lymphadenopathy. The chest is clear. The cardiac and abdominal exams are unremarkable. Complete blood count and chemistry panel are normal. A chest x-ray shows a cavity with surrounding infiltrate in the left upper lobe (Fig. 13.1).

Medical Microbiology for the New Curriculum: A Case-Based Approach, by Roberta B. Carey, Mindy G. Schuster, and Karin L. McGowan.
Copyright © 2008 John Wiley & Sons, Inc.

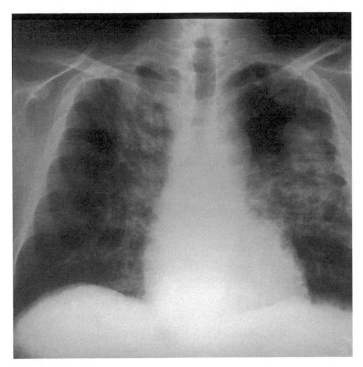

FIGURE 13.1 Chest x-ray showing cavity with surrounding infiltrate.

13.2. DIFFERENTIAL DIAGNOSIS

Infectious Causes

Bacteria

Actinomyces spp.

Anaerobic lung abscess (due to aspiration)

Mycobacterium tuberculosis (TB)

Mycobacterium other than *M. tuberculosis* (MOTT)

Nocardia spp.

Pseudomonas and other gram-negative rods (causes of cavitary bacterial pneumonia)

Rhodococcus equi

Viruses

Viruses are an unlikely cause of this chronic illness.

Fungi

Aspergillus spp. (aspergilloma)

Histoplasma capsulatum (rare)

Parasites

Dirofilaria spp.

Noninfectious Causes

Lung carcinoma

Sarcoid

Wegener's granulomatosis

CLINICAL CLUES

? Insidious onset of fever, cough, anorexia, and weight loss? Think pulmonary TB or malignancy. Bacterial pneumonia has an abrupt onset.

? Copious, foul-smelling sputum in a patient with poor dentition? Think anaerobic lung abscess. An air–fluid level in a cavity seen on x-ray would be further evidence of aspiration pneumonia.

? Negative skin test? This does not rule out TB since 25% of patients may have a false-negative reaction due to malnutrition or HIV.

? Is the patient HIV-positive? Think TB since patients with HIV are more likely to develop active tuberculosis.

13.3. LABORATORY TESTS

Although cavitary lesions may be caused by noninfectious conditions such as carcinoma, most such cavities result from infection. Infections due to mycobacteria including *M. tuberculosis*, various fungi, *Nocardia*, *Actinomyces*, *Rhodococcus equi*, anaerobes, and gram-negative rods, such as *Pseudomonas aeruginosa*, are capable of causing cavitary disease. The systemic fungi *Cryptococcus neoformans*, *Coccidioides immitis*, and *Histoplasma capsulatum* rarely cause cavitary pneumonia; however, it is a frequent finding in invasive pulmonary aspergillosis. Laboratory tests should include aerobic and anaerobic bacterial culture, Gram stain, mycobacterial culture and smear for acid-fast bacilli (AFB), and fungal culture and smear.

Sputum from a deep cough and not saliva must be submitted for bacterial aerobic culture, acid-fast culture, and fungal culture. Most laboratories will evaluate the quality of a sputum specimen using the Gram stain smear and will reject specimens for bacterial culture that contain more than 10 squamous epithelial cells per low-power magnification field (10×objective) because it represents oral secretions (Fig. 13.2). Because a multitude of anaerobes are normally present in sputum and upper respiratory secretions, a transtracheal aspirate or direct lung aspirate must be submitted for anaerobic culture.

Acid-fast organisms are so named because they stain well with basic dyes such as carbol–fuchsin or auramine and then completely resist decolorization even with acid–alcohol. The cell walls of mycobacteria contain long-chain fatty acids (mycolic acids), which bind basic dyes quite effectively but account for the inability of the mycobacteria to also stain

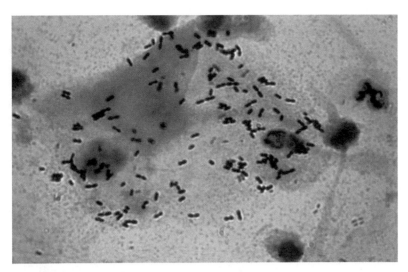

FIGURE 13.2 Sputum Gram stain showing unacceptable specimen quality.

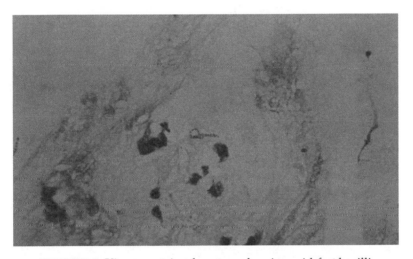

FIGURE 13.3 Kinyoun stain of sputum showing acid-fast bacilli.

with Gram stain. The Kinyoun stain (carbol–fuchsin), Ziehl–Neelsen stain (heated carbol–fuchsin), and Truant's stain (auramine–rhodamine) are all used to detect acid-fast organisms. With the Kinyoun and Ziehl–Neelsen stains, acid-fast-positive organisms stain bright red on a blue background using light microscopy (Fig. 13.3). With the auramine–rhodamine stain, acid-fast positive organisms stain a bright yellow or orange against a black background using fluorescent microscopy (Fig. 13.4). The auramine–rhodamine fluorochrome dyes are preferred by most laboratories because the technique is more sensitive and large areas of the smears can be examined under low-power microscopy. Mycobacteria appear as beaded, slender, and sometimes curved AFB-positive rods. It is not possible to distinguish the species of mycobacteria using the AFB smear. The

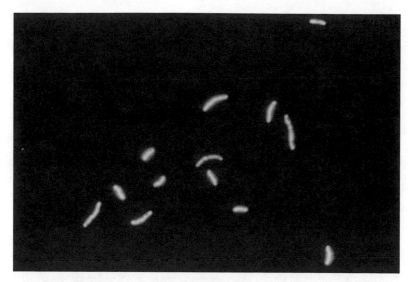

FIGURE 13.4 Auromine–rhodamine stain showing acid-fast bacilli.

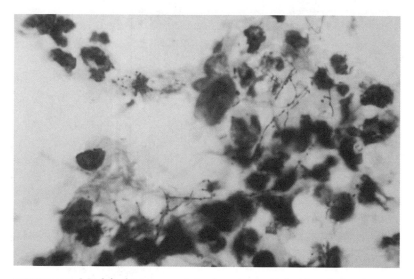

FIGURE 13.5 Modified Kinyoun stain showing acid-fast beaded rods compatible with *Nocardia* species.

overall sensitivity of an acid-fast smear is poor, ranging from as low as 20% to as high as 80% depending on the stage of illness and specimen type. For this reason, a negative AFB smear result does not rule out mycobacterial disease. Results of positive AFB smears are quantitated (+1 to +4), which is helpful in the initial evaluation of the patient as well as response to treatment. Acid-fast stains are not specific for mycobacteria. *Nocardia* are branching gram-positive rods that stain acid-fast when a milder decolorization step is used for the acid-fast stain (Fig. 13.5).

To rule out pulmonary mycobacterial infection, a total of three consecutive sputum specimens should be submitted for acid-fast culture and smear. First-morning expectorated sputum samples are considered the best specimens. If appropriately obtained sputum specimens are not diagnostic, then specimens obtained by bronchoscopy should be considered because the yield is higher (90%). In infants and children, first-morning gastric lavage specimens are the specimen of choice because young children frequently swallow their sputum. First-morning urine specimens for AFB smear and culture can also be obtained but are culture-positive in only a third of cases.

Definitive diagnosis, organism identification, and appropriate therapy of tuberculosis rely on the isolation of the organism. All specimens submitted for mycobacterial smear and culture are digested with strong acid or alkali to remove nonmycobacterial flora and are then concentrated to increase culture sensitivity. The traditional solid media available for mycobacterial culture include Lowenstein–Jensen (LJ) and Middlebrook (MB) agars. Because growth of *M. tuberculosis* can take 4–6 weeks on these traditional media, many labs now use broth media in combination with automated instruments to increase the sensitivity and decrease the time to detection. Mycobacteria grow more quickly in liquid than in solid media, and by using broth-based systems, *M. tuberculosis* can be recovered in as quickly as 8–10 days. Traditionally, identification of *Mycobacterium* spp. from positive cultures required the use of biochemical tests, which took as long as 2–3 weeks. Now, once growth in broth or on solid media is detected, rapid identification of *M. tuberculosis* complex, *M. avium* complex, *M. kansasii*, and *M. gordonae* can be accomplished using DNA probes. For identification of *M. tuberculosis*, DNA probes have yielded a sensitivity and specificity of ≥99%. For *Mycobacterium* spp. other than those identifiable by DNA probe, high-performance liquid chromatography (HPLC) or traditional biochemical tests are used for identification to species.

Nucleic acid amplification tests are now available for the diagnosis of *M. tuberculosis*. Because of their mycolic acid cell wall, the mycobacteria have shown themselves to be quite resistant to simple cell disruption and nucleic acid extraction techniques. In clinical specimens such as sputum, the detection limits using nucleic acid amplification have varied from as little as 100 to as many as 1000 organisms. For this reason, many laboratories have accepted only AFB-smear-positive sputum specimens from untreated patients for nucleic acid amplification testing. A number of nucleic acid amplification kits for *M. tuberculosis* have been FDA-approved, but their role in laboratory practice is still unclear. They will most likely be used in conjunction with AFB smear and *M. tuberculosis* culture for best results; however, at this time the use of nucleic acid amplification is not performed routinely because it is cost-prohibitive.

Two methods are used for susceptibility testing of mycobacteria: an agar-based method, which can take 2–3 weeks for completion; and a broth-based automated method, which takes 5–7 days to complete. Many hospital laboratories refer mycobacterial susceptibility testing to reference or state public health laboratories. All initial isolates of *M. tuberculosis* should be susceptibility-tested to first-line agents: isoniazid (INH), rifampin, ethambutol, and pyrazinamide (PZA) (See results in Table 13.1). Second-line agents for testing include amikacin, ciprofloxacin, cycloserine, ethionamide, kanamycin, *para*-aminosalicylic acid (PAS), and rifabutin.

TABLE 13.1.	Results of Susceptibility Testing of Our Patient's *M. tuberculosis* Isolate	
Drug	Minimal Inhibitory Concentration (MIC) (μg/mL)	Interpretation
Ethambutol	5.0	Susceptible
Isoniazid	0.1	Susceptible
Pyrazinamide	100	Susceptible
Rifampin	1.0	Susceptible

13.4. RESULTS

Because tuberculosis was in the differential diagnosis for this patient, a tuberculin skin test (Mantoux) was administered in the ED prior to admission. The Mantoux skin test is an intradermal injection of 0.1 mL of purified protein derivative (PPD), which is applied to the forearm and examined 48–72 h after injection. The result of the test is based on the diameter of induration at the injection site, and test interpretation varies with the patient's estimated risk for TB (e.g., healthy adult vs. young child vs. IV drug abuser vs. HIV-positive patient). This patient's skin test was determined to be positive when read at 48 h. Bacterial and fungal cultures were negative for pulmonary pathogens. Two of three auramine–rhodamine AFB smears were positive (+1) for acid-fast bacilli. AFB cultures performed using broth media were positive after 11 days of incubation. The Kinyoun stain of the broth culture demonstrated long cords of AFB, which is more typical of *M. tuberculois* (Fig. 13.6). The cultures were confirmed as *M. tuberculosis* by DNA probe.

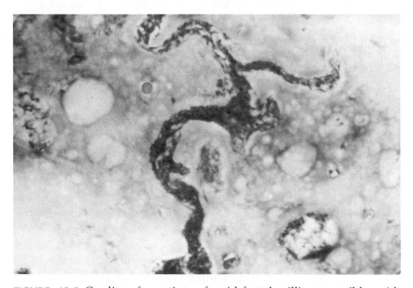

FIGURE 13.6 Cording formation of acid-fast bacilli compatible with *Mycobacterium tuberculosis*.

In the United States, all AFB-positive smears, positive mycobacteria cultures, and results of susceptibility testing must be reported to local and state departments of public health. This patient's smear, culture, and susceptibility testing results were reported as soon as each became available. In keeping with current guidelines, HIV testing was ordered on our patient to rule out a coinfection with this virus. Her serology test for HIV was negative.

13.5. PATHOGENESIS

Tuberculosis infections have been documented since the time of the Egyptian mummies in 2400 B.C. Despite the modern era of antibiotics, tuberculosis remains a killer of two million people worldwide each year. *M. tuberculosis* is spread person to person by aerosol droplets. Our patient may have acquired her infection from her grandmother, who had the "bad pneumonia." These tiny droplets bypass the defenses of the upper airway, such as cilia, and allow the organisms to lodge in the alveoli of the lungs. The organisms are disseminated by the lymphatics to the regional lymph nodes in the lungs, and at this time the TB skin test becomes reactive. In uncontrolled TB infections, the organisms destroy the lung by causing a caseous necrosis that has a cheesy consistency that retains the bacteria. The caseous necrosis progresses to a liquification state and releases the bacteria to disseminate into the bloodstream and then to the bones, joints, spleen, GI tract, and brain. This disseminated form of TB is called miliary TB.

M. tuberculosis survives and multiplies within inactivated macrophages. Activated macrophages can kill the organisms by eliciting a T helper cell (CD4+) and cytotoxic T-cell (CD8+) response. The CD4+ cells produce antibody and interferon gamma (IFNγ) that activates macrophages and stimulates endothelial cells to bind more T cells and attack infected tissues. The CD8+ cells kill infected phagocytes that have ingested the bacteria. Humoral antibody does not eliminate infection; it is T-cell immunity that ultimately leads to recovery and protection from reinfection with a new strain of TB.

If activated macrophages appear early in the infection, they can prevent damage to the lung. Macrophages fuse to form giant cells that combine with the T cells and other macrophages to produce a granulomatous response to wall off the growing lesion. This is known as a tubercle. The tubercles calcify, but microorganisms may survive in the tubercle during a period of latency and reactivate if the host cellular immunity wanes with cancer, HIV, or immunosuppressive therapy.

M. tuberculosis is a successful pathogen because it can multiply inside macrophages and monocytes and reduce the oxidative burst that would kill most bacteria within the cells. It also decreases the production of IL-12, a cytokine that stimulates a cell-mediated response. Mycobacteria produce compounds that interfere with T-cell activation, which is required to kill the bacterial cells. Ultimately, the growth of *M. tuberculosis* elicits an inflammatory response required to control infection, but with a price of extensive tissue damage.

13.6. TREATMENT AND PREVENTION

Antibiotics commonly used to treat bacterial infections are useless in treating tuberculosis. The routine first-line antituberculosis therapy includes a combination of isoniazid (INH), rifampin, ethambutol, and pyrazinamide. Treatment is required for a minimum of six months since the organisms grow slowly and it takes a long time to kill them. Combination therapy with multiple drugs is required since resistance to a single antibiotic occurs with high frequency. INH, the key antituberculosis agent, requires activation by catalase produced by the organism. A mutation in the catalase gene (*katG*) inactivates the catalase enzyme, resulting in resistance to INH.

Initial therapy is started with three or four antituberculosis drugs. Susceptibility testing may require 7–28 days after the organism is recovered in culture. Once the susceptibility pattern is known, a two-drug therapeutic regimen is common. If the patient's organism is susceptible to all antibiotics, as seen in our patient, the usual therapy is INH and rifampin, which are given for the entire 6 months of treatment with pyrazinamide during the initial two months. A patient suspected of having TB is put into respiratory isolation (a private room with negative pressure, and healthcare workers wear special protective masks, gowns, and gloves) until several specimens are reported as AFB smear negative. If the patient's smear is positive, the patient will remain in isolation until having received three days of antituberculosis therapy and is no longer considered to be highly infectious. The remaining months of treatment are given on an outpatient basis.

To ensure that patients are taking their medications, antituberculosis programs monitor patients undergoing their therapy. This is known as direct observed therapy (DOT). Completion of the full course of therapy is critical to protect the public health. Since the course of therapy is prolonged, patients tend not to comply over the long period of time. If they do not complete the course of therapy, the TB organisms that survive are usually resistant to the antibiotics they were taking, and they become infectious to others. Patients are recultured and smears performed after 3 months of therapy. If the smear is AFB-positive, drug-resistant TB should be considered. When TB treatment failure is suspected, two or more new drugs must be added while culture and susceptibility testing is in progress to ensure that the patient is being treated with more than one active agent.

Multidrug-resistant TB (MDR-TB) strains are defined as *M. tuberculosis* strains resistant to two or more antituberculosis agents. Patients with MDR-TB spread their infection for a longer period of time, and for those with infection there is a higher mortality rate. The W strain of TB in New York City was resistant to INH, rifampin, streptomycin, ethambutol, ethionamide, rifabutin, and kanamycin and was highly virulent and infective. Strains of MDR-TB are common in Russia, South Africa, and India. People migrating to the United States from these countries should be screened for infection from these resistant microorganisms. Extensively drug-resistant tuberculosis (XDR TB) is currently defined as *M. tuberculosis* that is resistant to isoniazid and rifampin, plus resistant to any fluoroquinolone and to at least one of three injectable "second-line" drugs (amikacin, kanamycin, or capreomycin). Because of the difficulty treating stains of XDR TB, the mortality rate is very high and spread of these organisms is a major public health concern.

People with a positive Mantoux skin test and no active tuberculosis disease are considered to have "latent" tuberculosis. To prevent the infection from progressing at a later time, therapy with INH is given for 9 months. At present there is no universally accepted vaccine against tuberculosis. Immunity requires a live vaccine to induce cellular immunity without causing harm to the recipient. A killed vaccine is ineffective. Vaccination with an avirulent strain of *M. bovis* (BCG), named for the researchers who found it, A. L. C. Calmette and C. Guérin, offers some protection to people who live in high-risk areas of the world. However, those vaccinated with BCG develop a reactive skin test so that a positive PPD is no longer a reliable means of detecting new infection. The effectiveness of BCG vaccination is controversial. It does not prevent reactivation in adults, and the efficacy rate varies. New candidate vaccines are a primary focus of tuberculosis research.

13.7. ADDITIONAL POINTS

- A number of demographic factors can increase a patient's risk for exposure to TB or to drug-resistant strains of TB. These include:
  - Having close contact with someone known or suspected to have TB
  - Caring for people who have untreated TB (healthcare professionals)
  - Living or working in high-risk settings (prisons, nursing homes, military barracks, or homeless shelters)
  - Having poor access to healthcare (homeless people, migrant farmworkers, people who abuse alcohol or drugs)
  - Traveling to or from regions where untreated TB is common, such as Africa, Asia (except Japan), Caribbean, eastern Europe, Latin America, and Russia
  - Having a condition that weakens or impairs the immune system [the elderly, newborns and young children, women who have recently given birth, patients receiving corticosteroid therapy, patients with human immunodeficiency virus (HIV/AIDS) infection, some cancers, or poorly controlled diabetes].

- The QuantiFERON® Gold-TB test (QFT) is a recently described serology test that measures IFNγ, a component of cell-mediated immunity to *M. tuberculosis*. The test is designed to replace tuberculin skin testing and has the advantage of being less affected by BCG vaccination. Unfortunately, once the blood samples are taken, they must be processed within 12 h, which is very impractical in most settings, and at this time, very few laboratories have experience with the assay. Just as with tuberculin skin testing, interpretation of QFT results is influenced by the patient's estimated risk for TB infection.

- In 1959, E. H. Runyon suggested a classification of the nontuberculous mycobacteria based on colony morphology, pigmentation, and growth rate. That classification is still in use today. Each group is briefly described in Table 13.2.

TABLE 13.2.	Runyon Classification of Nontuberculous Mycobacteria		
Runyon Group	Group Name	Description	Examples
I	Photochromogens	Colonies that produce pigment after a 1 h light exposure and take >7 days to grow on solid media	*M. kansasii*, *M. marinum*
II	Scotochromogens	Colonies that produce pigment in both the light and the dark and take >7 days to grow on solid media	*M. gordonae*, *M. scrofulaceum*
III	Nonphotochromogens	Colonies that do not produce pigment and take >7 days to grow on solid media	*M. avium*, *M. intracellulare*, *M. haemophilum*
IV	Rapid growers	Colonies that grow on solid media in ≤7 days	*M. fortuitum*, *M. chelonae*, *M. abscessus*

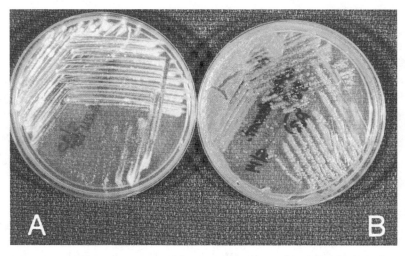

FIGURE 13.7 Photochromogen *Mycobacterium kansasii* before (A) and after (B) light exposure.

■ Growth of *M. kansasii* (Runyon group I) is shown in Fig 13.7 as yellow pigmented colonies after light exposure and nonpigmented colonies when grown in the dark. The orange pigmented colonies of *M. gordonae* (Runyon group II) are in contrast to the dry, buff colonies of *M. tuberculosis* (Fig. 13.8).

■ In addition to tuberculosis, HIV- infected patients have a high incidence of infection with *Mycobacterium avium-intracellulare* (MAI), which may be isolated from respiratory, blood, and stool specimens. Multiple antibiotics are required to treat MAI infections, and the antimicrobials used are not the same ones given for tuberculosis. HIV-infected patients may

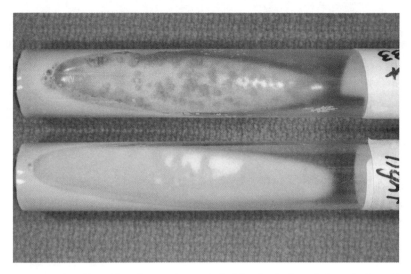

FIGURE 13.8 Growth of nonpigmented *Mycobacterium tuberculosis* and gold-pigmented *Mycobacterium gordonae* on Lowenstein–Jensen agar.

acquire infections with other unusual species of mycobacteria, such as *M. haemophilum*, and treatment varies according to the species of mycobacterium cultured.

■ Chronic pulmonary disease resembling tuberculosis has been associated with some nontuberculous mycobacteria. This occurs most frequently with *M. kansasii* and MAI. The disease occurs most often in the elderly, presenting in males as chronic obstructive pulmonary disease (COPD) and in females as chronic dilatation of the bronchi marked by paroxysmal coughing (bronchiectasis) and scarring.

■ *Mycobacterium marinum* prefers to grow at cooler temperatures (30°C) and causes skin lesions, especially on the hands of patients who handle fish and fish tanks.

■ *Dirofilaria* spp. are zoonotic filarial worms and are transmitted by mosquitoes. Diagnosis is achieved by microscopic identification on histologic sections of affected tissues such as lung. There are no serology tests for this parasite.

SUGGESTED READING

CAMPBELL, I. A. AND O. BAH-SOW, Pulmonary tuberculosis: Diagnosis and treatment, *Br. Med. J.* **332**:1194–1197 (2006).

CDC, Trends in tuberculosis—United States, 1998–2003, *MMWR* **53**:209–214 (2004).

CDC, Controlling tuberculosis in the United States, *MMWR* **54**(RR-12):1–81 (2005).

CDC, Guidelines for preventing the transmission of *Mycobacterium tuberculosis* in health-care settings, *MMWR* **54**(RR-17):1–141 (2005).

KATO-MAEDA, M. AND P. M. SMALL, User's guide to tuberculosis resources on the internet, *Clin. Infect. Dis.* **32**:1580–1588 (2001).

MYERS, J. P., New recommendations for the treatment of tuberculosis, *Curr. Opin. Infect. Dis.* **18**:133–140 (2005).

Student with Chronic Fever, Dry Cough and Pneumonia

14.1. PATIENT HISTORY

The patient is a 21 year-old college student who lives and goes to school in Delaware. He presents in early September to a local hospital with a 3-week history of fever with occasional chills, headache, myalgia, pleuritic chest pain, and nonproductive cough. He denied shortness of breath, but lost 10 lb over the past month. He reported no night sweats, or blood in his sputum. There were no known exposures to tuberculosis, but on further questioning he revealed that he had traveled extensively during the summer break. He spent the summer backpacking through the states of Ohio, Kentucky, Indiana, Illinois, and Missouri, and when he needed to earn additional spending money, he worked at construction sites. On physical exam (PE) he had a temperature of 38°C (100.4°F), pulse 126 beats/min, respirations 30 breaths/min, and blood pressure 110/70 mm Hg. He was well-appearing and in no acute distress but complained of intense fatigue. Chest exam revealed bilateral inspiratory pulmonary crackles. The remainder of his PE was within normal limits. A chest x-ray demonstrated bilateral patchy, nodular infiltrates and hilar lymphadenopathy (Fig. 14.1).

14.2. DIFFERENTIAL DIAGNOSIS

The relatively long duration of symptoms and nonproductive cough make common causes of community acquired pneumonia, such as *Streptococcus*

Medical Microbiology for the New Curriculum: A Case-Based Approach, by Roberta B. Carey, Mindy G. Schuster, and Karin L. McGowan.
Copyright © 2008 John Wiley & Sons, Inc.

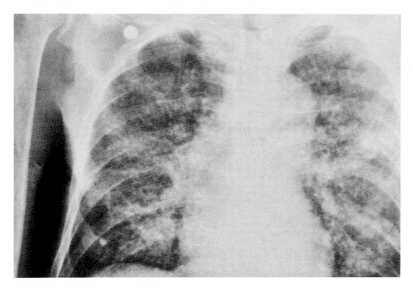

FIGURE 14.1 Chest x-ray with patchy infiltrates and hilar lymphadenopathy.

pneumoniae, less likely. This patient's presentation fits better for an atypical pneumonia. While this patient initially presented with nonspecific symptoms and signs of an acute respiratory illness, his x-ray findings, hilar lymphadenopathy, and weight loss now suggest a more chronic systemic illness. Agents capable of causing such a systemic illness include those listed below.

Infections Causes

Bacteria

Chlamydia pneumoniae

Chlamydia psittaci

Legionella pneumophila

Mycobacterium tuberculosis

Mycoplasma pneumoniae

Rickettsia

Coxiella burnetii (Q fever)

Fungi

Blastomyces dermatitidis

Coccidioides immitis

Histoplasma capsulatum

Penicillium marneffei

Pneumocystis carinii (jiroveci)

Parasites

Parasites are an unlikely cause of this systemic illness.

Viruses

Adenovirus

Influenza virus

Respiratory syncytial virus

Noninfectious Causes

Mediastinal granuloma

Sarcoidosis

Tumor

CLINICAL CLUES

? Have respiratory symptoms persisted for more than 14 days? Think atypical pneumonia rather than bacterial.

? Does patient have work or hobbies related to birds, bat exposure, or recent travel outside the usual living area? Histoplasmosis should be considered.

? A respiratory infection that does not respond to the course of antibiotics for community-acquired pneumonia? Routine bacterial infection less likely.

? Presence of mediastial lymph node enlargement? Commonly observed in tuberculosis and histoplasmosis.

14.3. LABORATORY TESTS

Routine laboratory testing that would be performed on this patient include a complete WBC count with differential, hemoglobin, platelet count, serum electrolytes, and a routine chemistry panel; bacterial and fungal blood cultures (10 mL blood each, ×2); microscopic examination of sputum for bacteria, acid-fast bacilli, fungi, and *Pneumocystis* sp.; routine bacterial, *Legionella,* fungal, and mycobacterial cultures (×3) of sputum; urine antigen testing for *Legionella* and *Histoplasma capsulatum*; and serology testing for *Mycoplasma pneumoniae, Chlamydia pneumoniae,* and *H. capsulatum.* Serology for *Chlamydia psittaci* is indicated if there is an exposure to birds, and for *Coxiella burnetii,* if there is a history of exposure to farm animals. Because of its superior recovery of endemic mycoses, such as *Histoplasma capsulatum,* the lysis–centrifugation (Isolator®) method should be used for fungal blood cultures.

While influenza virus is unlikely because of the time of the year, both respiratory syncytial virus and adenovirus can be seen year round. The laboratory diagnosis of either virus can be made by direct staining of respiratory tract secretions using fluorescent antibody (FA), membrane enzyme immunoassay (EIA) tests, conventional cell culture, shell vial culture, and serologic testing.

The fungi *H. capsulatum*, *Blastomyces dermatitidis*, *Coccidioides immitis*, and *Penicillium marneffei* are all found in well-defined geographic (also called endemic) zones. This patient's travel to the states of Ohio, Kentucky, Indiana, Illinois, and Missouri placed him well within the endemic zone for *H. capsulatum*. Because the natural habitat for the infective mould phase of *H. capsulatum* is soil, working in construction sites where the soil is constantly turned over and aerated would place him at increased risk of inhaling the spores and acquiring disease. Acute symptomatic histoplasmosis is diagnosed by fungal stains and microscopic examination of sputum, blood, or bone marrow, and deeper respiratory specimens such as pleural fluid (if present), BAL, or lung biopsy; by fungal culture; and by serology (both antigen and antibody testing). In patients with disseminated infection, culture of bone marrow may increase the yield.

14.4. RESULTS

Microscopic examinations of the pleural fluid for bacteria, acid-fast bacilli, and fungi were negative. Sputum submitted for bacterial, fungal, and mycobacterial culture was also negative; however, after 8 days of incubation, fungal blood cultures were positive for a mould presumptively identified as *H. capsulatum*. The regional public health laboratory later confirmed the isolate as *H. capsulatum*. In addition, both the immunodiffusion and complement fixation tests for antibodies were later reported as positive. Antigen detection testing performed on urine was negative. *H. capsulatum* can be diagnosed in the laboratory using a variety of methods, described below.

Microscopy/Histology

A presumptive and frequently early diagnosis of histoplasmosis can be made by the observation of small, intracellular, budding yeast in specimens such as lung tissue, BAL, sterile fluids, blood, and bone marrow aspirates (Fig. 14.2). The yeast can be seen when stained with standard stains such as Giemsa or hematoxylin and eosin or by special stains such as Gomori methenamine silver stain. This is the fastest way to make the diagnosis of histoplasmosis.

Culture

Definitive diagnosis of histoplasmosis requires isolation and identification of the organism by culture. Unfortunately, cultures may require as long as 4–6 weeks of incubation before becoming positive. The rate of positivity varies with the specimen type (blood and bone marrow best), the course of the disease (chronic pulmonary highest rate), and the immune status of the patient. Immunocompromised patients and those with HIV have a higher organism load. Cultures are most often positive in patients with disseminated or chronic pulmonary histoplasmosis with more than 3–4 weeks of symptoms. Like the other endemic fungi, *H. capsulatum* is

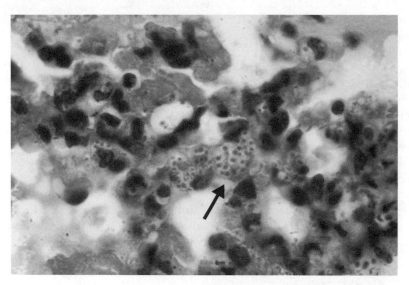

FIGURE 14.2 Giemsa stain of bone marrow showing small intracellular yeasts.

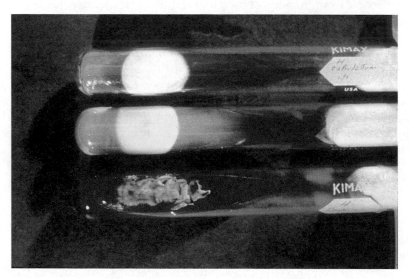

FIGURE 14.3 Culture tubes of *Histoplasma capsulatum* showing mould (top, middle) and creamy yeast (bottom).

dimorphic meaning it exists in two different physical forms (yeast and mould) depending on the incubation temperature (Fig. 14.3). The tiny yeast form is seen in clinical specimens and is grown in the laboratory on fungal media when incubated at 35°C. The mould form is found in the environment and grown in the laboratory when cultures are incubated at 25–30°C. Microscopic examination of the mould shows characteristic thick-walled macroconidia (spores) and small microconidia (Fig. 14.4), which are the infective spores that are inhaled. Isolation and observation of the typical mould stage is not considered sufficient to identify the isolate as *H. capsulatum*. Confirmation requires converting the mould form to the

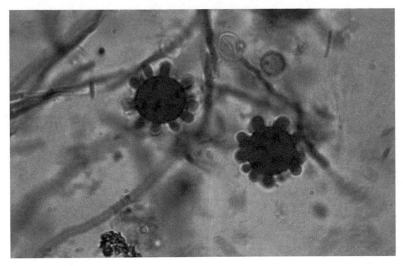

FIGURE 14.4 Microscopic image of *Histoplasma capsulatum* macroconidia.

yeast form or using molecular techniques to confirm the presence of specific ribosomal RNA. Because of this requirement, final culture results are often delayed.

Serology

The serologic diagnosis of histoplasmosis can be made using the immunodiffusion (ID) test, using the complement fixation test (CF), or by antigen detection. The CF test is more sensitive than the ID test and becomes positive 2–6 weeks after infection. A single titer of $\geq 1:32$ in a person not living in the endemic region or a twofold rise in titer between acute and convalescent serum specimens taken 3–4 weeks apart is considered strong evidence of infection. Because CF antibody levels can persist for years, paired acute and convalescent serum specimens are preferred. The ID test is less sensitive than the CF but more specific. Two major precipitin bands (M and H) can be detected with the ID test. In most cases (75%) of acute disease, the M band can be detected, but this band can persist for months after the infection. The H band is specific for acute disease but occurs in only approximately 20% of patients.

The histoplasma polysaccharide antigen (HPA) detection test can be performed on urine or serum using enzyme immunoassay (EIA) methodology. Measuring HPA is most helpful when diagnosing disseminated histoplasmosis, particularly in immunocompromised hosts who are incapable of generating detectable levels of antibodies. In such a population, sensitivities for the test range within 78–98% in urine and 60–88% in serum. In addition, with AIDS patients the HPA levels can be prognostic since the HPA level will drop as a result of successful therapy and increase if therapy fails. The HPA assay does not appear sufficiently sensitive in other forms of the disease, and studies have shown cross-reactions (false positives) in patients with paracoccidioidomycosis, blastomycosis, and with *P. marneffei*.

Molecular

PCR assays for the direct detection and identification of *H. capsulatum* from clinical specimens have been developed but are not yet available for diagnostic use.

14.5. PATHOGENESIS

H. capsulatum is the most common endemic mycosis in the United States and has recently emerged as an important opportunistic infection among HIV-infected persons living in regions where the organism is prevalent. In the United States most cases are seen in people living along the Ohio and Mississippi River valleys or visitors traveling to Central America and South America, where the organisms are endemic. *H. capsulatum* is found in bat feces (guano) and soil enriched with bird droppings, which enhance the growth and sporulation of this organism. Spores (microcondia) become airborne when contaminated soil is disturbed, and air currents can carry the organism to individuals far from the site of contamination. Exposure may occur during construction, renovation, or demolition of buildings, while cleaning areas contaminated with bird guano, or while exploring caves (spelunking). Person-to-person transmission through respiratory contact has not been reported for this disease.

In the lung, the inhaled microconida convert into yeasts. Macrophages phagocytize the yeasts but are unable to kill them. Instead, yeast-laden macrophages can disseminate the fungal organisms to the liver, spleen, bone marrow, and lymph nodes. Cellular immunity is essential in the defense against *Histoplasma*. Sensitized T lymphocytes combine with cytokines to convey fungicidal activity on the macrophages, which brings the infection under control in the immunocompetent patient.

Infection begins from about 10 days to 3 weeks after exposure. The severity of illness depends on the intensity of exposure and the immunity of the host. Asymptomatic infection or mild pulmonary disease follows a low-intensity exposure in healthy individuals. Heavy exposure may lead to severe diffuse pulmonary infection. The organisms can spread hematogenously to other organs, and granulomas may develop in the liver and spleen. Disseminated histoplasmosis is more likely to occur in the immunocompromised host, and central nervous system (CNS) disease occurs in 10–20% of these patients. High-risk groups include any immunocompromised person with decreased cellular immunity, especially those with cancer, post-transplantation, or HIV infection.

14.6. TREATMENT AND PREVENTION

Antifungal treatment is rarely indicated for the healthy person with acute pulmonary histoplasmosis. The disease is self-limiting in the immunocompetent host. If a fever persists for more than 3 weeks, it may indicate that the disease is progressing, and antifungal therapy may be required. Treatment with itraconazole for 6–12 weeks should be given to those who show no clinical improvement after 1 month of observation.

In patients with more severe manifestations who are sufficiently ill to require hospitalization, amphotericin B should be used. On release from the hospital, treatment can be continued with oral itraconzazole. Patients with chronic pulmonary histoplasmosis require long-term itraconazole therapy. Lifelong maintenance therapy is required to prevent relapse in patients with AIDS and histoplasmosis.

There is no proven prophylaxis to protect those at high risk for acquiring *H. capsulatum*. No vaccine is available to protect those living in endemic areas of the world.

14.7. ADDITIONAL POINTS

■ The three systemic mycoses found in the United States, histoplasmosis, blastomycosis, and coccidioidomycosis, have similar clinical presentations and can be acquired by inhalation of the fungal spores of the mould form of the organism. In addition, blastomycosis can be acquired by introduction of the organism into the skin following trauma. However, they have unique geographic distribution and morphology. A comparison of these dimorphic fungi highlights their identifying characteristics is presented in Table 14.1. The yeast phase and mould phase of

TABLE 14.1.	Comparison of Systemic Mycosis Characteristics		
Characteristic	Histoplasmosis	Blastomycosis	Coccidioidomycosis
Organism name	*Histoplasma capsulatum*	*Blastomyces dermatitidis*	*Coccidioides immitis*
Morphology at 37°C	2–4-μm intracellular yeasts (histiocytes, macrophages)	8–15-μm broad-based figure-8-shaped yeast	30–60-μm spherules filled with 2–5-μm endospores (no yeast phase)
Morphology at 30°C	Mould with spiny (tuberculated) macroconidia and oval-shaped microconidia	Mould with oval shaped microconidia	Mould with alternating barrel-shaped arthroconidia
Endemic zone	Ohio and Mississippi River valleys	North central and southeastern USA	Southwestern USA (California, Arizona, New Mexico) and northern Mexico
Habitat	Bat feces and soil contaminated by bird droppings	Decaying vegetation, soil contaminated with beaver excreta	Desert sand
Clinical	• Asymptomatic • Acute pneumonia • Chronic pneumonia • Disseminated disease (skin, bone marrow, CNS)	• Asymptomatic • Acute pneumonia • Cutaneous disease • Disseminated disease (skin, G/U tract, bones, CNS)	• Asymptomatic • Acute pneumonia • Disseminated disease (skin, bones, CNS; more likely in dark-skinned races, AIDS patients)

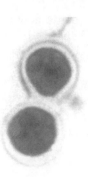

FIGURE 14.5 Microscopic image of *Blastomyces dermatitidis* broad-based budding yeasts.

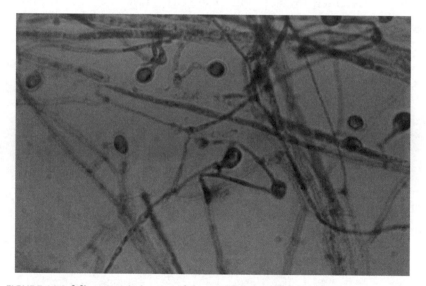

FIGURE 14.6 Microscopic image of the mould phase of *Blastomyces dermatitidis*.

Blastomyces are shown in Figs. 14.5 and 14.6. In tissue, *Coccidioides* takes the form of a spherule filled with endospores (Fig. 14.7), while in the environment it takes the mould form with alternating barrel-shaped arthroconidia (Fig. 14.8).

■ *H. capsulatum*, *B. dermatitidis*, and *C. immitis* share common antigens and cross-reacting antibodies in patient sera can make the interpretation of CF serology tests difficult.

■ Acute pulmonary histoplasmosis can mimic tuberculosis. Patients will often have cough, fever, and weight loss. Chest x-ray may show a

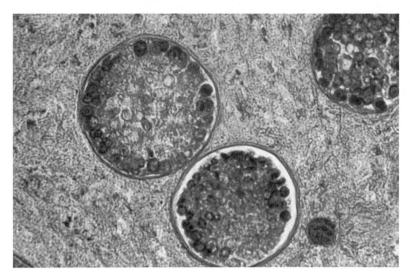

FIGURE 14.7 Spherules of *Coccidioides immitis* in tissue.

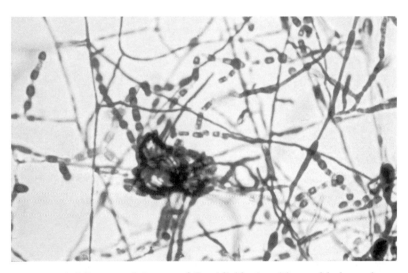

FIGURE 14.8 Microscopic image of *Coccidioides immitis* mould phase showing barrel-shaped arthroconidia.

miliary pattern indistinguishable from miliary tuberculosis. Patients with chronic pulmonary histoplasmosis can present like those with reactivation tuberculosis with cavitary pulmonary infiltrates.

■ The histoplasmin skin test is used for epidemiologic studies and is not used to diagnose acute disease. Skin test positivity cannot distinguish past from present infection.

■ *H. capsulatum* has recently been demonstrated to be transmissible by organ transplantation (cadaveric liver and kidney transplants), but the precise mechanism of transmission has not yet been defined.

SUGGESTED READING

PANACKAL, A. A., R. A. HAJJEH, M. S. CETRON, AND D. W. WARNOCK, Fungal infections among returning travelers, *Clin. Infect. Dis.* **35**:1088–1095 (2002).

WHEAT, L. J. Histoplasmosis: A review for clinicians from non-endemic areas, *Mycoses* **49**:274–282 (2006).

WHEAT, L. J., G. SAROSI, D. MCKINSEY ET AL., Practice guidelines for the management of patients with histoplasmosis, *Clin. Infect. Dis.* **30**:688–695 (2000).

Bone Marrow Transplant Recipient with Nodular Pneumonia

15.1. PATIENT HISTORY

The patient was a 45 year-old female with a history of acute myeloid leukemia for which she received an allogeneic bone marrow transplant (BMT) 4 months ago. Her course has been complicated by chronic graft-versus-host (GVH) disease with liver and skin involvement. Because of this, she has been treated with high-dose prednisone for the past 4 months. She now presents to the emergency department (ED) with a history of several days of fever, a nonproductive cough, and chest pain on inspiration (pleuritic chest pain). On physical exam (PE) she appeared mildly short of breath and coughed throughout the exam. Her temperature was 38.5°C (101.3°F), her pulse was 112/min, respiratory rate was 20/min, and blood pressure 110/70 mm Hg. Examination of the chest showed no evidence of consolidation, but a pleural friction rub was present on the right, anteriorly. Her pharynx was clear, her head and neck exam was within normal limits, and she had no lymphadenopathy. The remainder of her PE was unremarkable. She has no history of travel, pet contact, smoking, or allergies. Her chronic medications since BMT include tacrolimus (a drug that suppresses T-cell function), fluconazole, trimethoprim–sulfamethoxazole, and prednisone. A chest x-ray revealed bilateral patchy infiltrates. A chest computerized tomography (CT) showed bilateral nodular infiltrates with surrounding areas of hazy, "ground glass" opacification. She was admitted for further workup.

Medical Microbiology for the New Curriculum: A Case-Based Approach, by Roberta B. Carey, Mindy G. Schuster, and Karin L. McGowan.
Copyright © 2008 John Wiley & Sons, Inc.

15.2. DIFFERENTIAL DIAGNOSIS

The process of BMT can be divided into phases, each of which is characterized by specific host immune defects, and consequently each is associated with specific types of infections. Phase 1 is the pre-engraftment period (days 0–30) and includes the time from marrow infusion to marrow engraftment. During this period, the recipient's immune defect is a decrease in the number of neutrophilic leukocytes (neutropenia), and the predominant causes of infection during this stage are similar to those seen in any neutropenic host, namely, bacteria, *Candida* spp., and herpes simplex virus (HSV). If neutropenia persists for more than 2–3 weeks, patients are also at risk for *Aspergillus* and other mould infections. Phase 2 is the early recovery or post-engraftment period (days 30–100), and the immunodeficiency seen during this period is T cell in nature. Fungal and viral pathogens, particularly cytomegalovirus (CMV), predominate during this period. During this period patients are also at risk for *Pneumocystis carinii* (*jiroveci*) as well as severe infections with respiratory viruses (adenovirus, respiratory syncytial virus, parainfluenza, and influenza). Phase 3 is the late post-engraftment period (days >100) and is characterized by both B- and T-cell host defense defects. Bacterial infections due to encapsulated organisms, such as pneumococcus, and viral infections such as varicella zoster virus infection, are most common. In the subset of patients who require ongoing significant immunosuppression (those with chronic GVH disease), the risk for infection with *Aspergillus* and other moulds, as well as CMV and *Pneumocystis* is ongoing. Organisms causing pneumonia in bone marrow transplant recipients include those listed below.

Infectious Causes

Bacteria

> *Burkholderia cepacia*
>
> *Haemophilus influenzae*
>
> *Legionella* spp.
>
> *Mycobacterium tuberculosis*
>
> Mycobacteria other than *M. tuberculosis* (MOTT)
>
> *Nocardia* spp.
>
> *Pseudomonas* spp.
>
> *Staphylococcus aureus*
>
> *Streptococcus pneumoniae*

Fungi

> *Aspergillus* spp.
>
> *Candida* spp.
>
> Endemic mycoses (if recipient lived in areas of endemic histoplasmosis, coccidioidomycosis, or blastomycosis)
>
> *Fusarium* spp.

Pneumocystis carinii (*jiroveci*)

Rare causes: *Bipolaris, Cryptococcus neoformans, Curvularia, Mucor* spp., *Penicillium* spp.

Parasites
Toxoplasma gondii

Viruses
Adenovirus

Cytomegalovirus (CMV)

Epstein–Barr virus (EBV)

Herpes simplex virus (HSV)

Human herpesvirus 6 (HHV-6)

Influenza virus

Parainfluenza virus

Respiratory syncytial virus (RSV)

Varicella zoster virus (VZV)

Noninfectious Causes
Diffuse alveolar hemorrhage

Graft versus host disease (GVH)

Malignancy

CLINICAL CLUES

? Does the patient have decreased T-cell function? Think fungal or viral infection in patients with decreased cellular immunity.

? Does the patient have decreased B-cell function? Think bacterial infection in patients with decreased humoral immunity. For at least a year after BMT, patients have impaired B-cell immunity and respond poorly to vaccines. They are at risk for infections with encapsulated organisms, such as *Streptococcus pneumoniae*.

? Presence of a halo or air crescent sign on the chest CT? These signs have a high association with aspergillus infection. Clinical clues to invasive pulmonary aspergillosis include fever, pleuritic chest pain, hemoptysis, and the presence of a pleural friction rub.

15.3. LABORATORY TESTS

A wide variety of specimens should be collected for detecting the various pathogens that cause disease in BMT recipients. Blood and urine specimens should be submitted for bacterial, fungal, and viral cultures. At least two

10-mL samples of blood collected from separate sites should be taken. For patients with signs and symptoms of pulmonary disease, sputum should be collected for Gram stain, bacterial and fungal cultures, and direct fluorescent antibody (DFA) stain and culture for *Legionella* spp. Urine should also be submitted for *Legionella* antigen testing. With transplant patients who are neutropenic, the laboratory should be alerted to withhold applying sputum screening criteria to evaluate the quality of the specimen. A minimum of three separate first-morning sputum specimens should be submitted for acid-fast stain and mycobacterial culture.

A bronchoalveolar lavage (BAL) is considered a more reliable and accurate specimen than sputum when diagnosing pulmonary infections in BMT and solid organ recipients. For this reason, BAL specimens are extensively studied by both microbiology and pathology with a battery of tests. This should include smears and cultures for aerobic bacteria, fungi, mycobacteria, viruses, *Legionella* spp., *Nocardia* spp., and *Pneumocystis carinii* (*jiroveci*). Histologic and immunologic stains are available for *P. carinii*, *Toxoplasma gondii*, and various fungi. If pulmonary nodules are present, lung biopsy of the nodules is also a superior specimen and should be evaluated by both microbiology and pathology with a battery of tests similar to those performed on a BAL specimen. Special stains to detect fungi and *P. carinii* should always be requested in the initial evaluation of BAL and/or tissue specimens.

Fungal infections in BMT recipients can be detected by isolation of the organism (i.e., culture), antigen detection, and histopathology. A methodology called lysis-centrifugation (Isolator®) enhances the recovery of fungi, particularly the endemic mycoses, from blood. While the method is very labor-intensive and expensive, its use with immunosuppressed patients can be justified because of its superior recovery of filamentous fungi. The exception is *Aspergillus* spp., which are rarely recovered from blood cultures. Calcofluor white is a whitening agent that binds to cellulose and chitin in the cell walls of fungi. When portions of specimens are mixed with calcofluor white and viewed with a fluorescent (FA) microscope, fungal cells and hyphae are more easily visualized than on Gram stain. Many microbiology laboratories perform a calcofluor white stain rather than Gram stain when specimens are submitted for fungal workup. Antigen tests for *Cryptococcus neoformans* (serum) and *Histoplasma capsulatum* (serum and urine) are useful for the early diagnosis of either pathogen. Use of polymerase chain reaction (PCR) to diagnose aspergillosis or other fungal diseases is still investigational with false-positive and false-negative results being reported.

Viral infections in BMT recipients can be detected by culture, antigen detection, histologic examination of tissue, and PCR. CMV can be detected early with direct antigen detection assays. Both CMV and HSV can be detected rapidly using PCR. Culture methods combining shell -vial techniques and immunofluorescent staining can also provide a rapid diagnosis with CMV, HSV, and VZV, which are common opportunists in BMT recipients. Adenovirus, influenza virus, parainfluenza virus, and RSV can be detected by direct FA staining and immunofluorescent microscopy. In addition, viral culture should always be ordered.

Other initial laboratory tests should include a complete blood count with differential, hemoglobin, hematocrit, and platelet count; serum glucose, blood urea nitrogen (BUN), creatinine, sodium, potassium, chloride, carbon dioxide, total protein, albumin; and liver function studies.

15.4. RESULTS

High-resolution computerized tomography (CT) is one of the best tools for diagnosing pulmonary aspergillosis. A chest CT performed on this patient when she was seen in the ED was significant because it showed bilateral nodular infiltrates with surrounding areas of hazy, "ground glass" opacification. This is called a "halo sign" and is suggestive of early-stage pulmonary aspergillosis (Fig. 15.1). Later-stage aspergillus disease shows a crescent sign on CT, which is an air crescent located near the periphery of a lung nodule caused by the contraction of infarcted tissue (Fig. 15.2). Both signs are highly suggestive of invasive pulmonary aspergillosis specifically in BMT recipients, but not diagnostic. Because of the suggestive CT findings, a BAL was immediately performed on this patient, and a calcofluor white smear performed on the specimen was positive for septate hyphae. Gomori methenamine silver and PAS stains performed on the BAL specimen were also microscopically positive for 45° angle (dichotomous) branching, septated, nonpigmented hyphae suggestive of *Aspergillus* spp. (Fig. 15.3). Two days later, fungal and bacterial cultures were positive for *A. fumigatus* (Figs. 15.4, 15.5).

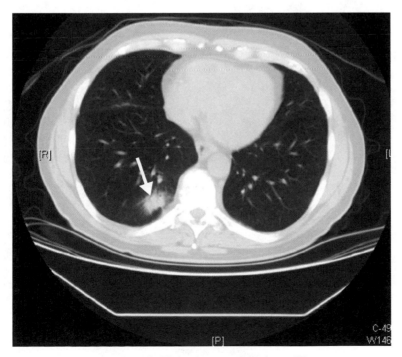

FIGURE 15.1 Halo sign seen on chest CT.

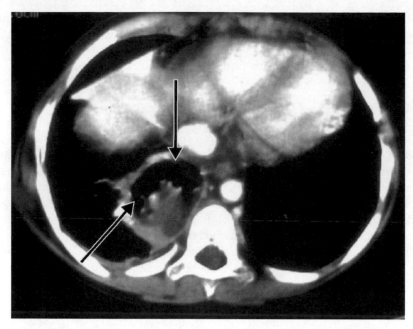

FIGURE 15.2 Air crescent sign seen on chest CT.

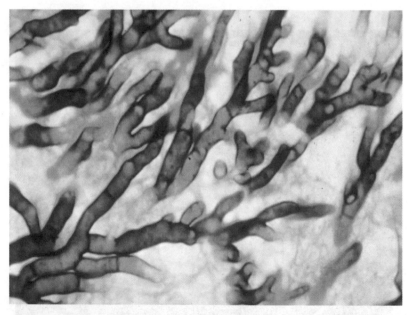

FIGURE 15.3 Dichotomous (Y-shaped) branching and septate hyphae compatible with aspergillosis.

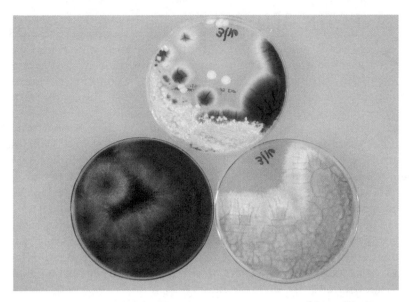

FIGURE 15.4 *Aspergillus* species growing on various culture media.

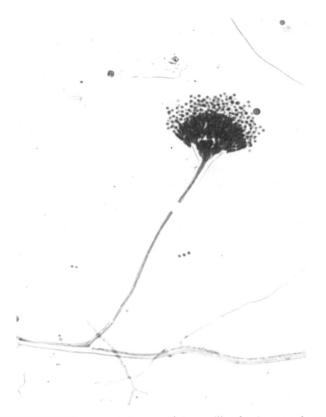

FIGURE 15.5 Microscopic image of *Aspergillus fumigatus* colony.

15.5. PATHOGENESIS

A. fumigatus is a saprophytic mould whose spores can be found world-wide in the soil and air. *Aspergillus* spp. can be introduced into the body by trauma to the skin and deeper tissues, but it is most commonly acquired by inhaling the spores (conidia) into the respiratory tract. The concentration of fungal conidia increases in settings where soil is being disrupted by strong wind currents or during construction projects. Environmental sampling indicates that humans inhale several hundred *A. fumigatus* conidia daily. Exposure to aspergillus can lead to allergic aspergillosis, colonization with the organism, or tissue invasion. Invasive aspergillosis is uncommon in immunocompetent individuals; however, it causes a devastating disease in the immunosuppressed patient. Neutropenia or neutrophil dysfunction and long-term corticosteroid therapy are the most common predisposing factors for invasive aspergillosis. Other risk factors include cytotoxic chemotherapy, bone marrow or organ transplant, and congenital or acquired immunodeficiency. The number of immunosuppressed patients has risen dramatically since the mid-1990s, and *A. fumigatus* is currently the most prevalent airborne fungal pathogen. Our patient received an allogeneic BMT, which puts her at higher risk for invasive aspergillosis than those who receive autologous bone marrow.

Alveolar macrophages form the first line of defense against the inhaled conidia, which elude the protective cilia in the upper airway and allow the organism to reach the alveoli of the lung. If the number of macrophages is decreased or their activity is dysfunctional, the conidia can germinate into hyphael forms of the mould that can invade tissue. The presence of hyphae activates complement and produces chemotaxic factors that elicit a neutrophil response. Hyphae are the primary target for the activated neutrophils. The fungus can combat the host response by producing complement inhibitors, proteases, and mycotoxins. The infection progresses across tissue planes by invasion of blood vessels, which results in infarction and tissue necrosis, a hallmark of invasive aspergillosis. Specific proteins, called adhesins, allow the conidia to bind to the membrane- associated host proteins. Adherence is essential before the fungus can penetrate the tissue and kill the phagocytic cells that protect the host. Other virulence factors include hemolysins to lyse the erythrocytes, antioxidants to obstruct killing by the phagocytic cells, and the natural pigment of the conidia that inhibits phagocytosis.

Pulmonary infection is usually manifested in the immunocompromised patient by fever that is unresponsive to broad-spectrum antibiotic therapy, although patients on long-term, high-dose corticosteroids may not always have elevated temperatures as a sign of infection. Chest pain, cough, and blood in the sputum (hemoptysis) may occur. The patient may have a chest x-ray with patchy, nodular infiltrates or one with normal findings. A CT scan is more likely to detect pulmonary changes. The infection may progress beyond the lungs into the liver, spleen, and kidney. The organism can spread from the sinuses into the brain (rhinocerebral aspergillosis), which manifests as mental status changes and lethargy or coma. Infection of the heart valves (endocarditis), the cornea (keratitis), deeper tissues of the eye (endophthalamitis), or skin may occur in the immunocompromised host.

15.6. TREATMENT

Because invasive aspergillosis is highly lethal in the immunocompromised host, therapy must be initiated when there is a suspicion of the diagnosis, even without definitive evidence. Despite appropriate antifungal therapy, mortality of invasive aspergillosis exceeds 80% in patients with neutropenia. Treatment must include reversal of the underlying predisposing condition, as well as medical and surgical therapy. In our BMT patient, engraftment of the new bone marrow is vital to the control of her disease and recovery from the infection. Administration of immune stimulating factors, such as granulocyte colony stimulating factor (G-CSF), may increase the fungicidal activity of neutrophils, but it is not routinely recommended in these patients.

Historically, the major antifungal drug has been amphotericin B, which targets the ergosterol production required for the fungal cell membrane. This antifungal agent has nephrotoxic side effects and lacks activity against some *Aspergillus* species. Newer classes of antifungal agents, such as voriconazole, an azole that inhibits cytochrome P450 required for cell membrane synthesis, and caspofungin, an echinocandin that inhibits glucan synthesis required for the cell wall, are having better success in treating serious aspergillus infections. Other new azole compounds, posaconazole and ravuconazole, are showing promise in treating invasive aspergillosis with fewer side effects than traditional amphotericin B therapy. Prophylaxis with micofungin, a newer echinocandin, is ongoing, and results may prove effective in preventing invasive disease.

In some patients, antifungal therapy can be discontinued when the neutrophil count increases to >500 cells/mm^3. However, if the patient requires subsequent cytotoxic chemotherapy, antifungal therapy must be restarted. Surgical debridement of infected sinuses or skin tissue may be required in addition to the administration of antifungal therapy. Our patient received a lipid preparation of amphotericin B for 3 weeks, followed by one month of voriconazole. Her corticosteroids were successfully tapered without flare-up of her GVH disease, and eventually, she recovered.

While in the hospital, the use of positive pressure rooms with air being filtered by high-efficiency particulate air filters (HEPA) may protect the neutropenic patient from early infections. However, most infections occur after the patient is released from the hospital and is being followed in the outpatient setting.

15.7. ADDITIONAL POINTS

■ An aspergillus antigen assay that tests for galactomannan in patient serum using enzyme-linked immunosorbent assay (ELISA) has recently been FDA-approved for diagnosing invasive aspergillosis. In BMT recipients tested twice weekly, galactomannan detection exhibited a sensitivity of 94% and a specificity of 99%. This test performs best when serial specimens rather than a single specimen from a patient can be tested.

■ In contrast to the 45° angle branching, septated, nonpigmented hyphae seen with *Aspergillus* spp., the *Zygomycetes* (*Mucor, Absidia, Rhizopus*)

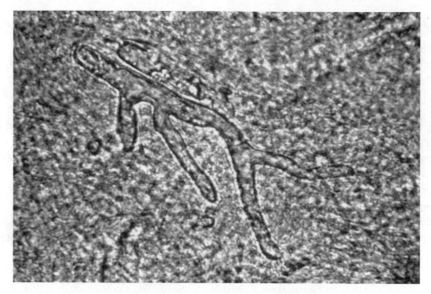

FIGURE 15.6 KOH preparation showing nonseptate hyphae.

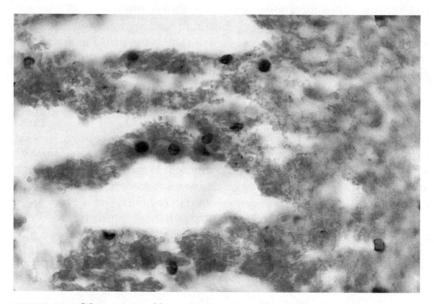

FIGURE 15.7 Silver stain of bronchial aspirate showing cells of *Pneumocystis carinii*.

produce wide, nonseptate, nonpigmented hyphae with 90° angle branching when seen microscopically (Fig. 15.6).

■ The laboratory diagnosis of *P. carinii* pneumonia is based on the direct and/or histologic examination of BAL or tissue specimens. The trophozoite and cysts forms of the organism stain with calcofluor white, Giemsa, or Gomori-methenamine silver stains (Fig. 15.7). Monoclonal antibodies attached to a fluorescent dye that allow for rapid and direct

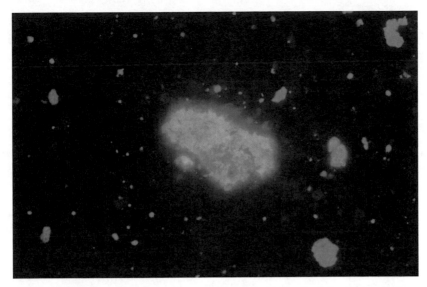

FIGURE 15.8 Positive fluorescent antibody stain for *Pneumocystis carinii*.

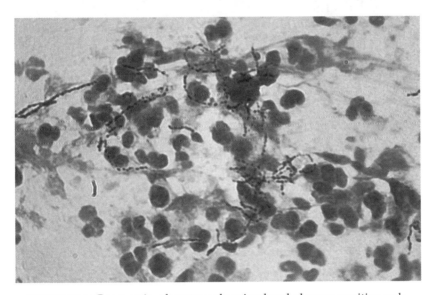

FIGURE 15.9 Gram stain of sputum showing beaded gram-positive rods.

fluorescent microscopic examination of specimens are also available (Fig. 15.8). The organism does not grow in culture, serology is not useful, and PCR methods are still investigational.

■ *Nocardia* spp. are branching gram-positive rods that are partially acid-fast (AFB) (Figs. 15.9, 15.10). *Nocardia* spp. and *Rhodococcus* spp. are aerobic, and although these organisms grow on routine bacterial culture media, they may require 3–4 days of incubation. Both groups cause pulmonary disease in BMT recipients.

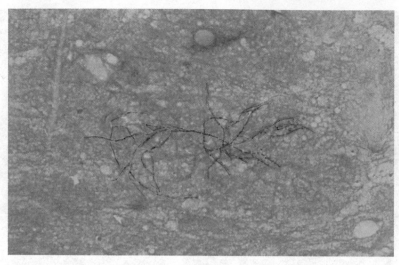

FIGURE 15.10 Modified Kinyoun stain showing branching acid-fast rods typical of *Nocardia* species.

SUGGESTED READING

LaRocco, M. T. and S. J. Burgert, Infection in the bone marrow transplant recipient and role of the microbiology laboratory in clinical transplantation, *Clin. Microbiol. Rev.* **10**:277–297 (1997).

Latge, J. P. *Aspergillus fumigatus* and aspergillosis, *Clin. Microbiol. Rev.* **12**:310–350 (1999).

Maertens, J., J. V. Eldere, J. Verhaegen et al., Use of circulating galactomannan screening for early diagnosis of invasive aspergillosis in allogeneic stem cell transplant recipients, *J. Infect. Dis.* **186**:1297–1306 (2002).

Stevens, D. A., V. L. Kan, M. A. Judson et al., Practice guidelines for diseases caused by *Aspergillus, Clin. Infect. Dis.* **30**: 696–709 (2000).

Boy with Acute Fever, Headache, and Confusion

16.1. PATIENT HISTORY

A previously healthy 16 year-old male was transported to a local emergency department (ED) after presenting to his high school nurse with fever, severe headache, vomiting, and confusion. He said that he began to feel ill the day before, and denied taking any illegal drugs or having any head injury from playing sports or trauma. On physical exam he was uncomfortable-appearing, drowsy but arousable, lying with his eyes closed, and lethargic. His temperature was 40°C (104°F); his blood pressure 120/80 mm Hg; pulse, 80/min; and respiratory rate, 14 breaths/min. His neck was somewhat rigid, and he complained of pain when his head was bent forward (anterior flexion). His initial skin exam revealed no rash. Later, when a spinal tap (lumbar puncture) was being performed, scattered nonraised purplish round red spots caused by intradermal hemorrhage (petechiae) appeared on his back, trunk, and legs (Figs. 16.1, 16.2).

16.2. DIFFERENTIAL DIAGNOSIS

High fever and drowsiness in this patient suggests a systemic neurologic event, which could be caused by any of the following:

■ Meningitis—an inflammation of the meninges, which, are the three membranes that cover the brain and spinal cord

Medical Microbiology for the New Curriculum: A Case-Based Approach, by Roberta B. Carey, Mindy G. Schuster, and Karin L. McGowan.
Copyright © 2008 John Wiley & Sons, Inc.

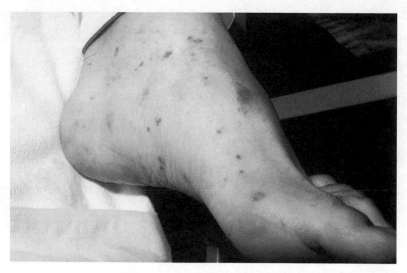

FIGURE 16.1 Petechiae on foot.

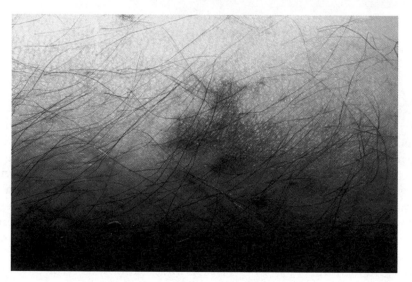

FIGURE 16.2 Close-up of petechiae on skin.

- Encephalitis—an inflammation of the brain
- Thrombosis—such as cavernous sinus thrombosis
- Brain abscess
- Brain lesion
- Trauma—subdural hematoma
- Tumor
- Subdural empyema—an accumulation of pus in the outermost membrane that covers the brain (dura mater)
- Drugs

The presence of a stiff neck suggests meningitis as the most likely diagnosis. The patient's vomiting may be a sign of elevated intracranial pressure.

Patients with fever and neurologic signs receive a complete neurologic examination as well as a general physical exam. Vital signs may show a decreased blood pressure and elevated heart rate. The exam should include a careful search for any skin lesions, as petechiae or purpura are often seen in meningococcal infection. Photophobia and neck stiffness (nuchal rigidity) should be looked for as well. Unless contraindicated, a lumbar puncture (LP) is quickly performed to aid in the diagnosis of meningitis. From the LP, cerebrospinal (CSF) opening pressure, protein, glucose, and WBC count values are obtained and can be used to create a CSF meningitis profile. Various CSF profiles are listed in Table 16.1. Please keep in mind that no single abnormal value can stand alone as a predictor when examining the CSF profile. In patients with elevated intracranial pressure, a lumbar puncture may be contraindicated because of the risk of CNS extension of the brain through the foramen magnum (herniation). Patients with elevated intracranial pressure often have either a focal neurological exam or swelling of the optic disk (papilledema). Other contraindications for LP include focal neurologic signs, severe cardiorespiratory instability, bleeding disorder, and low platelet count (thrombocytopenia).

Infectious Causes

Specific agents associated with acute meningitis in a normal host include those listed below.

Bacteria
Escherichia coli and other enteric gram-negative rods

Haemophilus influenzae

Listeria monocytogenes

Neisseria meningitidis

Staphylococcus aureus

Streptococcus agalactiae (group B strep)

Staphylococcus spp., coagulase-negative

Streptococcus pneumoniae

Streptococcus spp. other than group B and *S. pneumoniae*

Viruses
Arbovirus

Enterovirus

Herpes simplex virus

Mumps virus (rare)

Parasites
Acanthamoeba spp.

Naegleria fowleri

Fungi and Mycobacteria
These agents cause chronic rather than acute meningitis.

TABLE 16.1. **CSF Meningitis Profile**

Infection Type	CSF Parameters (Normal Values)			
	Opening Pressure (80–100 mm H$_2$O)	WBCs (Average <5 Cells/mm^3)	Glucose ($^2/_3$ of serum glucose)	Protein (<40 mg/dL)
Bacterial (untreated)	Elevated	50–20,000 PMNs predominant	Low (often <25 mg%)	Elevated (150–1000)
Viral	Slightly elevated	50–1000 Lymphocytes predominant	Normal	Elevated slightly (<150)
Fungal, M. tuberculosis, or treated bacterial	Elevated	50–1000 Lymphocytes/monocytes (PMNs in 10% of TB meningitis)	Low	Elevated (300–600)
Listeria or parameningeal focus (brain abscess)	Elevated	Increased Lymphocytes	Normal	Normal or slightly elevated

Risk Factors

The LP results reported to the ED on our case patient revealed an elevated opening pressure; 1304 WBCs with 92% PMNs, 5% bands, and 3% monocytes; glucose 30 mg% (serum 100 mg%); and protein 143 mg/dL. This young man has acute bacterial meningitis.

Today the majority of cases of bacterial meningitis in children and adults are due to *S. pneumoniae* and *Neisseria meningitidis*; however, the age of the patient and the presence of underlying disease are major factors when attempting to predict the organisms responsible for acute bacterial meningitis. Considering those factors, the most likely causes of bacterial meningitis include those listed below.

Neonates (Infants < 6 Weeks of Age)
S. agalactiae (group B streptococcus), *E. coli* and other enteric gram-negative rods, *L. monocytogenes*, *S. pneumoniae*, *N. meningitidis*, *H. influenzae*.

2 Months–5 Years
S. pneumoniae, *N. meningitidis*, *H. influenzae*.

5–16 Years
S. pneumoniae, *N. meningitidis*.

Adults
S. pneumoniae, *N. meningitidis*, *S. aureus*, *L. monocytogenes*, *H. influenzae* (rare cause).

Elderly (>60 Years)
S. pneumoniae, *N. meningitidis*, *E. coli*, and other enteric gram negative rods; *L. monocytogenes*, *S. aureus*, *Streptococcus* other than group B, *H. influenzae* (rare cause).

Immunocompromised Patients
L. monocytogenes, *Pseudomonas aeruginosa*, enteric gram-negative rods (like *E. coli, Klebsiella*), fungi, *S. aureus*, coagulase-negative staphylococci, *Acinetobacter*, and anaerobes. In this group of patients, any organism has the potential to be a pathogen and should not be disregarded as a contaminant.

CLINICAL CLUES

? Rapid onset of fever and headache? Bacterial meningitis can progress in a few hours, especially meningococcal meningitis and pneumococcal meningitis.

? Are skin lesions present, especially at pressure sites like the belt line or under elastic bands? Minute (1–2 mm) hemorrhages into the skin or mucous membranes (petechiae) or larger (1–2 cm) subcutaneous hematomas (ecchymoses) are important clues in the diagnosis of meningococcal disease.

? Is the headache severe? Patients with severe headaches are more likely to have bacterial meningitis than viral meningitis.

16.3. LABORATORY TESTS

Other than the cell count, glucose, and protein analysis performed on the CSF specimen, CSF Gram stain and cultures for bacteria and viruses are critical tests to perform when making the diagnosis of meningitis. Blood cultures should always be obtained on any patient who is febrile. Other initial laboratory tests should include a WBC count with differential, hemoglobin, hematocrit, and platelet count; serum glucose (which should be taken as close to the time as the LP as possible for comparison with the CSF glucose), blood urea nitrogen (BUN), creatinine, sodium, potassium chloride, carbon dioxide, total protein, albumin, and liver function studies. If present, scrapings of petechial lesions should be obtained for Gram stain and culture. For best results, petechial lesions should be scraped until bleeding occurs.

Ideally, the LP should be performed at the same time that empiric antibiotics are started. Treatment for suspected meningitis should never be delayed for diagnostic purposes, given the high morbidity and mortality associated with a delay in antibiotics.

CSF specimens are collected using a LP kit that contains skin drapes, anaesthetic, Betadine (povidone iodine), syringe, needle, and four plastic sterile screwcapped tubes. The site should be disinfected with Betadine, and the needle (with stylet) inserted at the L3–L4, L4–L5, or L5–S1 interspace. On reaching the subarachnoid space, the stylet should be removed and CSF collected. A minimum of at least 1 mL of CSF should be placed into each of the four sterile tubes. One tube will be used for bacterial Gram stain and culture, one for cell count and differential, and one for CSF glucose and protein analysis, and the fourth one should be used for viral culture or saved at $-70°C$ for future use. In at least one of the collection tubes, larger amounts of CSF should be obtained whenever possible because if fungal or mycobacterial cultures are anticipated, larger volumes of CSF (5–10 mL) will be necessary for adequate testing. If insufficient CSF is obtained on the initial LP, follow-up LPs may be necessary. CSF should be transported to laboratories rapidly (<15 min), and testing of CSF should be performed as quickly as possible. CSF specimens for bacterial, fungal, or parasitic testing should be kept at room temperature (RT) during transport for ≤ 2 h if necessary. CSF for viral analysis should be kept on ice during transport or refrigerated.

Once received in the microbiology laboratory, CSF is centrifuged and the sediment is used for Gram stain and culture. Concentrating the CSF by cytocentrifugation before Gram staining increases the ability to detect 1000–10,000 bacterial cells/mL of CSF. If no antibiotics are given before the LP, the sensitivity of the Gram stain is about 92%. Media used routinely when performing bacterial cultures of CSF include 5% sheep blood agar, chocolate agar to grow bacteria with complex nutritional needs, and an enrichment broth to detect small numbers of bacteria (Fig. 16.3). Bacterial colonies on the agar plates or turbidity in the enrichment broth indicate the presence of microorganisms, which are Gram-stained, and the results are reported immediately. Microorganisms are further identified and antibiotic susceptibility testing performed. If no organisms are recovered, a final report can be expected in 3–5 days. Routine bacterial culture of CSF does

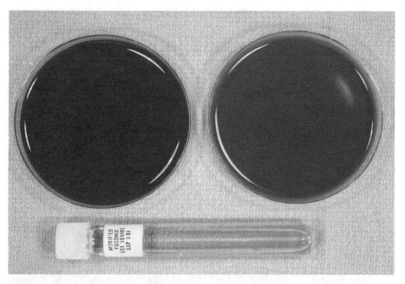

FIGURE 16.3 Blood agar, chocolate agar, and enrichment broth used to culture CSF.

not include culture for strict anaerobes since anaerobic bacteria rarely cause bacterial meningitis.

16.4. RESULTS

Gram stain of the petechial lesions as well as a cytocentrifuged Gram stain of CSF revealed many WBCs and moderate intracellular and extracellular gram-negative diplococci (Fig. 16.4). After overnight incubation, culture

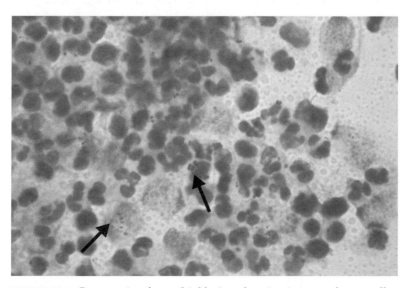

FIGURE 16.4 Gram-stain of petechial lesion showing intra- and extracellular gram-negative diplococci.

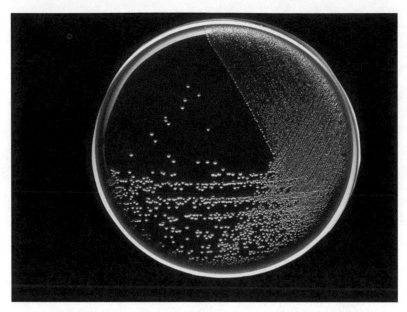

FIGURE 16.5 Colonies of *Neisseria meningitidis* on blood agar.

plates from blood, CSF, and skin specimens revealed nonhemolytic gray to white colonies on chocolate and sheep blood agars (Fig. 16.5). Since the bacteria are growing on both blood and chocolate agars, the bacteria are not *H. influenzae*, which would grow only on chocolate agar since this organism requires hemin (X factor) and NAD (V factor). *N. meningitidis*, *Moraxella catarrhalis*, and saprophytic *Neisseria* species (see Table 16.2) all grow well on both blood and chocolate agars, and all appear as gram-negative diplococci microscopically. In addition, they are all positive for the oxidase biochemical test (Fig. 16.6). They can be biochemically distinguished using rapid fermentation sugars, nitrate reduction, and a DNAse test.

The patient's isolate was biochemically identified as *N. meningitidis* by its ability to ferment both glucose and maltose (Fig. 16.7). *N. meningitidis* is encapsulated by polysaccharides and can be categorized into 13 serogroups; however, systemic disease is caused by five specific serogroups: A, B, C, Y, and W-135. Agglutination testing with specific

TABLE 16.2. **Biochemical Reactions for Identification of *Neisseria* Species and *Moraxella***

Organism	Fermentation Sugars			Nitrate Reduction	DNAse
	Glucose	Maltose	Lactose		
N. meningitidis	(+)	(+)	−	−	−
N. gonorrhoeae	(+)	−	−	−	−
M. catarrhalis	−	−	−	(+)	(+)

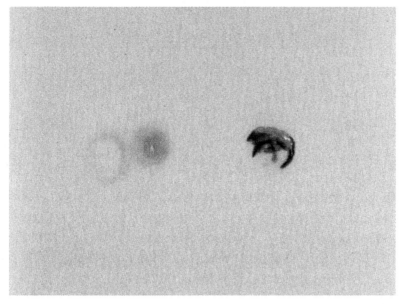

FIGURE 16.6 Oxidase test, negative (left), positive (right).

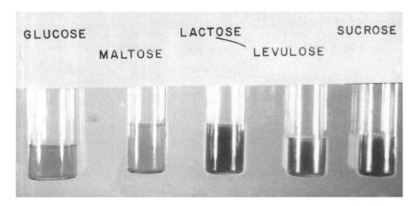

FIGURE 16.7 Carbohydrate fermentation tests (glucose- and maltose-positive).

group antisera revealed this patient's isolate to be *N. meningitidis*, group C, the serogroup seen most frequently in older children, adolescents, and adults. In general, antibiotic susceptibility testing is not routinely performed on *N. meningitidis* isolates; however, isolates should be routinely tested for β-lactamase production. β-Lactamase is an enzyme that is capable of breaking the β-lactam ring, a key structural part of antibiotics such as penicillin, ampicillin, and cephalosporins. Production of this enzyme confers resistance to the entire class of β-lactam antibiotics. The chromogenic cephalosporin test is used to detect β-lactamase production. When bacterial colonies are placed onto the surface of a disk containing cephalosporin substrate, a deep pink color is produced if the β-lactam ring is broken (Fig. 16.8). This patient's isolate was β-lactamase-negative.

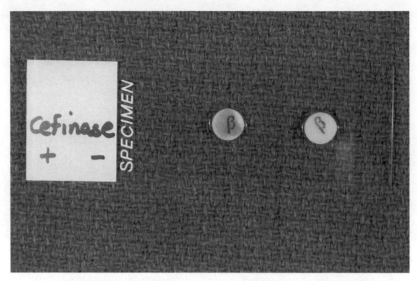

FIGURE 16.8 Cefinase disk test for β-lactamase production (positive, left; negative, right).

16.5. PATHOGENESIS

There are three phases in the process of developing acute bacterial meningitis: (1) colonization by the pathogen, (2) invasion of the CNS, and (3) the host's response to infection.

The initiation of bacterial meningitis begins as the host acquires a new organism by nasopharyngeal colonization. Pathogens possess specialized components, such as polysaccharide capsules, pili, and enzymes to allow adherence of organisms to nonciliated nasopharyngeal epithelium and establish mucosal colonization. Immunoglobulin A1 (IgA1) protects the upper respiratory tract by inhibiting the adherence of bacteria and preventing penetration into mucosal tissue. Meningeal pathogens (*N. meningitidis, H. influenzae, S. pneumoniae*) secrete metalloproteases that destroy IgA1, which facilitates the adherence of the bacteria to the host cells. A preceding viral infection of the respiratory tract decreases ciliated cells and increases the risk of invasive disease. Prior infection with influenza A promotes acquisition and colonization of bacterial pathogens, especially *H. influenzae* type b; hence the species name of the bacteria, which may follow infection with the influenza virus.

Pili of *N. meningitidis* allow adherence of the bacteria to the nasopharyngeal epithelial cells. Following attachment to specific cell receptors, the meningococci are transported in vacuoles across the nonciliated columnar epithelial cells. *N. meningitidis* is maintained in nature by colonizing the nasopharynx of humans. One-third of adults may carry *N. meningitidis* in their nasopharynxes, and 1–4% of infants and young children are also carriers. A positive nasopharyngeal culture in a healthy child does not mean that they are ill with this organism; however, they may spread the bacteria to others by contact with their respiratory secretions. If those exposed lack meningococcal antibody, they may become ill with the organism.

In the second phase, bacteria enter the bloodstream once the mucosal barrier has been compromised. The blood–brain barrier maintains the microenvironment of the CNS by restricting entry of pathogens, cells, and macromolecules, such as antibiotics. Bloodborne pathogens must cross the blood–brain barrier to invade the CNS. Bacteria may disrupt intercellular endothelial connections or invade white blood cells. Monocytes act like "Trojan horses" by carrying bacteria into the CSF across the choroid plexus. Alternatively, nonhematogenous invasion of the CSF by bacteria may occur when the barrier surrounding the brain is compromised by trauma, neurosurgery, sinusitis, mastoiditis, or otitis media. Once in the subarachnoid space, the bacteria multiply easily since the subarachnoid space lacks the white cells, complement, and antibody to destroy them.

Bacterial encapsulation is important for the organisms to survive in the bloodstream. Many of the major pathogens that enter the CNS are encapsulated. The capsule prevents phagocytosis by white cells and complement mediated killing. *N. meningitidis* has 13 antigenic varieties of polysaccharide capsule, but serogroups A, B, C, Y, and W-135 are those most commonly associated with human infections. Serogroup A is known as the epidemic type that is responsible for large outbreaks of meningococcal infections in sub-Saharan Africa. Serogroups B and C are most commonly found in the United States. Antibody to each individual serogroup protects the person from future infection only from that specific serogroup and does not offer protection against the others. Anticapsular antibody erases the protective mechanism of the polysaccharide capsule and allows phagocytosis by the polymorphonuclear leukocytes and macrophages. Likewise, activation of the alternative complement pathway counteracts the antiphagocytic activity of the capsular polysaccharide. Those with impairment of the alternative complement pathway have a higher frequency of meningitis. For example, patients who have been splenectomized and those with sickle cell disease have increased incidence of pneumococcal infections, and patients with deficiencies in terminal complement components (C5–C9) are prone to meningococcal infections.

In the third phase, replication and autolysis of bacteria in the CSF releases bacterial components, such as the lipopolysaccharides of gram-negative bacteria and the teichoic acid and peptidoglycan of gram-positive bacteria. Endotoxin is a powerful virulence factor that is released during the growth and lysis of meningococci. These bacterial surface components stimulate the release of host proinflammatory components of interleukins 1 and 6 (IL-1, IL-6), and tumor necrosis factor (TNF). These host factors are classified as hormone-like proteins (cytokines) that trigger a cascade of inflammatory mediators, which correlate with increased morbidity and mortality. Marked inflammatory response in the subarachnoid space is responsible for the negative consequences of bacterial meningitis. Inflammatory cells obstruct the outflow of the CSF from the subarachnoid space to the major sinuses and lead to interstitial edema, and eventually, to hydrocephalus. Thrombosis of the cerebral blood vessels results in infarction of the brain tissue.

Release of endotoxin into the circulatory system causes microvascular thrombosis, leading to the lack of perfusion of blood to the extremities (shock) and subsequent endothelial damage, resulting in petechiae. These hemorrhagic skin lesions are the hallmark of meningococcal disease, reflecting a vasculitis mediated by endotoxin and cytokines. The skin lesions can increase in size and number, progressing to disseminated intravascular coagulation (DIC), which occurs in all organs of the body, especially the adrenal glands. Overwhelming adrenal hemorrhage is known as Waterhouse–Friderichsen syndrome, and patients with severe DIC have a poor prognosis for recovery. Our patient did have petechial skin hemorrhages but did not progress to DIC because he received appropriate and timely medical attention.

On the upside, antibiotics cross into the CSF at a greater rate once the blood–brain barrier has been disrupted, so that some antibiotics that would not be active in the CNS are now able to achieve effective concentrations at this site. The downside is that antibiotic therapy contributes to host cell damage by rapidly lysing the bacteria and releasing their cell wall products. High concentrations of TNF released into the CSF by the host are associated with a worse outcome in the patient. The disease presentation that characterizes acute bacterial meningitis is a combination of bacterial invasion and host counterattack that damages tissues and causes long term sequelae, such as hearing loss and neurological deficits.

16.6. TREATMENT AND PREVENTION

Initially our patient was treated with a third-generation cephalosporin, ceftriaxone, and the glycopeptide, vancomycin. Third-generation cephalosporins cover most of the common bacterial agents that cause acute meningitis, but they do not effectively inhibit *L. monocytogenes*, which is resistant to all cephalosporins. In addition, some strains of *S. pneumoniae* have higher MICs to penicillin and cephalosporins due to altered penicillin-binding proteins (PBPs). Since the possibility of infection with penicillin-resistant pneumococci is high, vancomycin was added to the empiric regimen.

Once the pathogen in our patient was identified as a β-lactamase-negative *N. meningitidis*, our patient was given intravenous penicillin, the antibiotic of choice for treatment of systemic meningococcal disease. Because *N. meningitidis* strains with relative resistance to penicillin have been reported from many countries, there is some concern about the susceptibility of meningococci to penicillin. In the United States, the mechanism of relative resistance to penicillin involves the production of altered forms of one of the penicillin-binding proteins. While treatment with penicillin is still effective against these relatively resistant strains, there is evidence that low-dose treatment regimens can fail. Rare strains of meningococci produce a β-lactamase. These strains are more commonly found in Spain and Portugal, so, depending on the travel history, a person may be more likely to have an isolate with higher MICs to penicillin that would preclude this drug from being an effective antibacterial agent.

In addition to the antibiotic therapy, dexamethasone may be administered, either before or in conjunction with the antibiotic, to counteract the side effects of the cytokines produced by the host in response to the bacterial products. Dexamethasone treatment can attenuate the CSF inflammatory response associated with the administration of bacteriolytic antibiotics and decrease the neurologic sequelae.

When the pathogen is identified as *N. meningitidis*, the patient's family and close contacts should be given chemoprophylaxis. Among family members of a primary case of *N. meningitidis* meningitis, there is a 1000-fold higher risk of acquiring a secondary case when compared to nonfamily members. Contacts that reside in the same dwelling (house, dormitory, or barracks) and those who have close respiratory contact, such as family, boyfriend or girlfriend or those in daycare with the patient, should receive either oral rifampin, intramuscular (IM) ceftriaxone, or oral ciprofloxacin. Those who do *not* need chemoprophylaxis are their classmates, teammates, or hospital personnel, unless they have had close contact with the respiratory secretions of the index case.

In addition to chemoprophylaxis, there is a quadrivalent vaccine available for *N. meningitidis* groups A, C, Y, and W-135. Immunoprophylaxis is recommended for close contacts of an index case, and for military recruits, college freshmen who will be staying in dormatories, those traveling to high-risk areas, such as pilgrims going to Saudi Arabia for the Hajj, research or laboratory personnel who are routinely exposed to solutions of *N. meningitidis*, and for those with underlying diseases, such as terminal complement deficiency, asplenia, and alcoholics. Protective antibody is usually achieved within 7–10 days of vaccination. There is no effective vaccine against *N. meningitidis* group B. Attempts at preparing a vaccine of this group-specific polysaccharide have resulted in a poorly immunogenic preparation that offered little protection against meningococcal disease.

16.7. ADDITIONAL POINTS

- Bacterial meningitis is one of the top 10 infectious causes of death worldwide, and about half of the survivors have neurologic deficits and other sequelae after they recover from the initial infection.

- In the past, the peak age of risk for meningitis was 6–8 months when the protective maternal IgG antibodies disappeared. As a result of the effectiveness of the vaccine against *H. influenzae* type b, the median age for bacterial meningitis has risen from 15 months of age to 25 years of age, and *N. meningitidis* has become the leading cause of bacterial meningitis in children and young adults in the United States.

- Bacterial meningitis has a high mortality rate (>20%) in older adults despite modern antibiotic therapy. In this population more variable clinical presentations are seen, with fewer patients manifesting classic symptoms of high fever, stiff neck, and headache. Similarly, newborns and young infants present with irritability and failure to feed, without the typical stiff neck. Because of the increased intracranial pressure, the area over the bones in the skull that have not fused together may project outward in infants less than 1 month of age. This sign is known as a "bulging fontanelle."

- Administration of antibiotics prior to LP seldom significantly affects the CSF cell counts, protein, or glucose, but can reduce the yield of Gram stain and culture.

- Bacterial antigen tests to detect the unique capsular polysaccharides of the common agents that cause bacterial meningitis should not be ordered unless there is an abnormal cell count in the CSF (>5 cells/mL), and the CSF glucose concentration is below normal and the CSF protein concentration is above normal. Latex agglutination tests are commercially available for *S. pneumoniae*, *S. agalactiae* (group B), *H. influenzae* type b, and *N. meningitidis* groups A, B, C, Y, and W-135. Bacterial antigen tests are most helpful clinically when the patient has been treated with antibiotics prior to developing meningitis, and when culture is negative 24–48 h after incubation. Use of bacterial antigen tests is controversial because studies have shown these tests to be no better than Gram stain. Given the poor positive predictive values of CSF antigen tests, many labs have discontinued their use.

- Brudzinski and Kernig signs are two signs of meningeal irritation and are part of a physical exam. For the Kernig sign, with the patient supine, the hip and knee on one side are flexed to a 90° angle, and then, while keeping the hip immobile, one attempts to extend the knee. When meningeal irritation is present (positive Kernig), the attempt to extend the knee is resisted, causing pain in the hamstring muscles. When meningeal irritation is present (positive Brudzinski), the attempt to flex the patient's neck while the patient is supine causes involuntary flexion of the hips and knees.

- While petechiae are most often associated with *N. meningitidis* infections, other organisms such as *S. pneumoniae*, other streptococci, *H. influenzae*, *Acinetobacter* spp., coxsackievirus, and echovirus type 9 have also been associated with petechiae.

- Infection of CSF shunts is usually caused by organisms indigenous to the skin, such as coagulase-negative staphylococci, *S. aureus*, and *Propionibacterium* spp., or by gram-negative rods belonging to the *Enterobacteriaceae* (enteric gram-negative rods). In addition to agar plates, the fluid from a shunt is cultured in an enrichment broth, which increases the yield by 25%. Unlike the CSF in bacterial meningitis, shunt infections may not demonstrate a positive Gram stain of the CSF.

- Swimming in brackish ponds may expose a healthy person to ameba, such as *Naegleria fowleri*, which resides in these waters as part of the ecosystem. Inhalation of the contaminated water allows the ameba to enter the sinuses and gain access to the CNS, where it can cause rapidly progressive meningitis that is not treatable with the customary antibiotics. The CSF profile seen with *Naegleria* resembles that observed with bacterial meningitis.

SUGGESTED READING

CDC, Prevention and control of meningococcal disease, *MMWR* **49**(RR-07): 1–10 (2000).

CHAVEZ-BUENO, S. AND G. H. MCCRACKEN, JR., Bacterial meningitis in children, *Pediatr. Clin. N. Am.* **52**:795–810 (2005).

SINNER, S. W. AND A. R. TUNKEL, Antimicrobial agents in the treatment of bacterial meningitis, *Infect. Dis. Clin. N. Am.* **18**:581–602 (2004).

VAN DE BEEK, D., J. DE GANS, A. R. TUNKEL, AND E. F. WIJDICKS, Community-acquired bacterial meningitis in adults, *N. Engl. J. Med.* **354**: 44–53 (2006).

VAN DEUREN, M, P. BRANDTZAEG, AND J.W.M. VAN DER NEER, Update on meningococcal disease with emphasis on pathogenesis and clinical management, *Clin. Microbiol. Rev.* **13**: 144–166 (2000).

Woman with Lymphocytic Meningitis

17.1. PATIENT HISTORY

The patient is a 34 year-old Caucasian female who presents to the emergency department (ED) complaining of severe headache, vomiting, muscle aches (myalgias), and neck stiffness. Five days prior she had a sore throat and diffuse myalgias, but because she was on summer vacation with her family, she chose to take aspirin and wait. Six hours prior to presentation, her headaches became more severe and she began to complain of photophobia and a stiff neck. On physical exam (PE) she was a mildly ill-appearing woman sitting in a darkened treatment room complaining of headache. Her temperature was 38.5°C (101.3°F), blood pressure 110/80 mm Hg, pulse 120/min, and respiratory rate 20 breaths/min. Her neck was mildly stiff, and she had negative Kernig and Brudzinski signs. The remainder of her PE was within normal limits, including a neurology exam. She has not taken antibiotics; however, significant family history is that she has two children at home, both receiving antibiotics (amoxicillin) for streptococcal pharyngitis.

While this patient's symptoms are much less severe than those of Case 16, and she has no neurological deficits, a lumbar puncture is still warranted to aid in the diagnosis of meningitis. The results of a lumbar puncture performed in the ED revealed a slightly elevated opening pressure, 1100 WBCs with 60% lymphocytes, 35% polymorphonuclear neutrophils (PMNs), and 5% monocytes; CSF glucose of 60 mg% (serum glucose

Medical Microbiology for the New Curriculum: A Case-Based Approach, by Roberta B. Carey, Mindy G. Schuster, and Karin L. McGowan.
Copyright © 2008 John Wiley & Sons, Inc.

90 mg%); and protein 68 mg/dL. CSF Gram stain result: moderate WBCs, no organisms seen.

17.2. DIFFERENTIAL DIAGNOSIS

The term aseptic meningitis defines a syndrome of acute meningitis with WBCs present in the CSF and the absence of evidence of a bacterial pathogen. While this patient's CSF culture may eventually grow bacteria, initial CSF Gram stain results and the CSF profile information available in the ED would lead one to believe that she will meet the definition of aseptic meningitis. Additionally, most bacterial causes of meningitis result in a predominance of granulocytes in the CSF as opposed to viral etiologies, which result in a CSF lymphocytic pleocytosis. Infectious causes of aseptic meningitis include those listed below.

Infectious Causes

Bacteria

Borrelia burgdorferi (Lyme disease)

Leptospira spp.

Mycoplasma pneumoniae

Partially treated bacterial meningitis

Parameningeal focus (such as epidural abscess), which can cause inflammatory CSF response with negative cultures

Treponema pallidum (syphilis)

Viruses

Arboviruses: eastern and western equine encephalitis viruses, St. Louis, LaCrosse, West Nile

Cytomegalovirus (CMV)

Enteroviruses: enterovirus, coxsackievirus, echovirus, and poliovirus

Epstein–Barr virus (EBV)

Herpes simplex virus (HSV)

Human immunodeficiency virus (HIV)

Lymphocytic choriomeningitis virus (LCM)

Mumps

Varicella zoster virus (VZV)

Rickettsiae

Rickettsia rickettsii (Rocky Mountain Spotted Fever)

Parasites

Echinococcus granulosus

Plasmodium spp.

Taenia solium

Toxocara cati or *T. canis* (visceral larval migrans)

Fungi

Most often cause a more chronic meningitis with symptoms lasting weeks to months

Mycobacteria

Mycobacterium tuberculosis

Noninfectious Causes

Drug-induced/chemical meningitis [caused by NSAIDS (nonsteroidal antiinflammatory drugs)]

Carcinomatous or lymphomatous meningitis (patients often have cranial nerve abnormalities)

CLINICAL CLUES

[?] Has the patient had symptoms for 2–3 days? The course of viral meningitis is slower and more indolent than that of bacterial meningitis.

[?] What is the season of the year? Arboviruses and enteroviruses are endemic in the summer and early fall in the United States.

[?] Does the patient have a history of any sexually transmitted disease (HIV, HSV, syphilis) or genital lesion? Think acute HIV infection with aseptic meningitis, especially if rash, pharyngitis, and lymphadenopathy are present.

[?] Exposure to wooded areas or history of tick bite? Think Lyme disease or rickettsial diseases, such as Rocky Mountain Spotted Fever.

17.3. LABORATORY TESTS

The initial laboratory tests suggested in Case 16 would still be appropriate with this case: CSF Gram stain and cultures for bacteria and viruses as well as blood cultures. Whenever possible, all specimens should be taken prior to the administration of antibiotics. The CSF profile for this patient as well as the negative Gram stain, less severe symptoms, lack of prior antibiotic therapy, and absence of rash suggest viral meningitis, and the season of the year (summer or fall) would specifically favor enteroviruses. CSF for viral culture and other viral analysis should be placed into a sterile leakproof container and kept on ice during transport or refrigerated. The CSF should not be frozen, and CSF should not be placed in a viral transport medium because it would needlessly dilute the specimen.

Because many viruses replicate and are shed in body sites other than the CSF, it is appropriate to collect these specimens for viral culture as well as CSF in cases of suspected aseptic meningitis. Blood, stool, urine,

TABLE 17.1.	Collection and Transport of Specimens for Viral Tests		
Specimen	Virology Test	Collection Container	Transport Conditions
CSF	PCR	Leakproof, sterile container	4°C or on ice
CSF, urine, or stool	Culture	Leakproof, sterile container	4°C or on ice
Oropharynx or tissue	Culture	Viral transport medium	4°C or on ice
Urine	PCR	Leakproof, sterile container	Room temperature
Plasma or Serum	PCR	Heparinized, EDTA, red-, or gold-topped tube (5 mL)	Room temperature
Serum	Serology	Red- or gold-topped tube (5 mL)	Room temperature

pharynx, and in some cases brain tissue specimens are appropriate additional specimens for many of the viruses that cause aseptic meningitis. Specimens should be collected during the acute phase of the illness. If serology testing is anticipated, both acute and convalescent (3–4 weeks later) blood samples should be collected. See Table 17.1 for collection and transport guidelines.

For viral culture, once received in the laboratory, the specimens are inoculated onto a battery of appropriate cell culture lines. The presence of some viruses is suggested by a characteristic morphologic change that they cause in the cells, called cytopathic effect (CPE) (Figs. 17.1, 17.2). CPE can be seen as early as 24 h and as late as 23 days post-inoculation. Isolated viruses are then identified using specific monoclonal antibodies, neutralization assays, or hemadsorption.

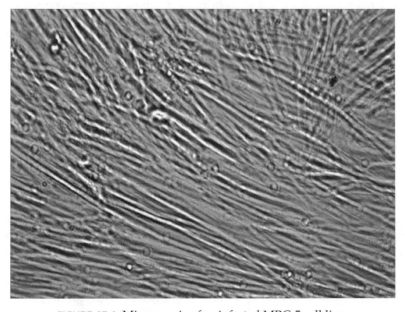

FIGURE 17.1 Microscopic of uninfected MRC-5 cell line.

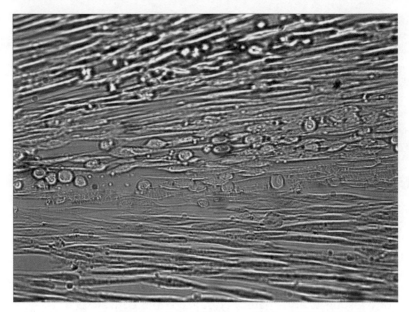

FIGURE 17.2 Cytopathic effect (CPE) from HSV on MRC-5 cell line.

While a wide variety of viruses can cause meningitis, almost 90% of cases are caused by enteroviruses. For both enterovirus and herpes simplex virus, use of the polymerase chain reaction (PCR) has proved to be superior to viral culture, and PCR is now the most rapid and accurate laboratory method to detect both viruses in CSF. Besides CSF, PCR for enteroviruses can also be performed on urine, plasma, body fluids, and tissue specimens.

Because the differential diagnosis of aseptic meningitis is extensive, additional laboratory testing is extremely dependent on information obtained from a carefully taken history and physical exam. The season of the year, travel to endemic areas, and other critical clues will suggest and justify additional laboratory testing.

17.4. RESULTS

CSF PCR for enterovirus was positive in the case patient within 48 h after the initial specimen was submitted to the laboratory. Most enteroviruses take 4–8 days to grow, and in this patient both stool and pharynx specimens were positive by viral culture; however, the CSF culture was negative.

17.5. PATHOGENESIS

Our patient has aseptic meningitis, which is an infection of the central nervous system (CNS) with meningeal inflammation, lymphocytic pleocytosis, and the absence of any bacterial pathogen in the spinal fluid cultures. Aseptic meningitis is most commonly caused by a virus as in this case, but other microorganisms can cause this disease, such as *Mycobacterium tuberculosis*, *Leptospira* spp., and *Borrelia burgdorferi* (Lyme disease). The

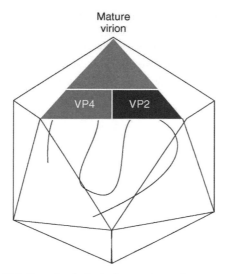

FIGURE 17.3 Icosahedral viral structure of an enterovirus.

infectious agent responsible for this young adult's illness is an enterovirus, a member of the *Picornaviridae*, which is the group of the smallest RNA viruses. The picornavirus family includes enteroviruses that are found in the human throat and lower intestinal tract, and the rhinoviruses that cause the common cold and are isolated from the nose and throat. The enteroviruses are named for their ability to infect intestinal tract epithelium and lymphoid tissues and to be shed into the feces. Traditionally enteroviruses were classified into coxsackieviruses A and B; polioviruses 1, 2, and 3; and echoviruses. In the 1960s newly discovered enteroviruses received a numeric designation (e.g., enterovirus 68) instead of being assigned to one of the traditional groups. Molecular typing methods have been used to identify new enteroviruses, and echoviruses 22 and 23 have been reclassified into a new genus named *Parechovirus*.

The enteroviruses have a genome of single-stranded positive sense RNA (ssRNA) that can act as its own messenger RNA (mRNA) and a capsid shell of 60 subunits with four major polypeptides (VP1,2,3,4) in an icosahedral formation (Fig. 17.3). Unlike the rhinoviruses, enteroviruses are resistant to acid (pH 3.0) for several hours, which allows them to survive the acid environment of the stomach and duodenum, and they can multiply efficiently at 37°C. Since the enteroviruses lack a lipid envelope, they are resistant to ether, as well as 70% alcohol, detergents, and 5% Lysol. Therefore, they can remain infectious in the environment for a period of time.

Humans are the natural host for polio viruses, coxsackieviruses, and echoviruses. Other enteroviruses are found in animals, but may not pass from animals to humans readily. Transmission is person to person by direct or indirect fecal–oral contact. Transmission may occur by the respiratory route since early in the infection, the virus replicates in the upper respiratory tract. The incubation period is usually 2–10 days, and it is common for concurrent infections to occur in the same family since secondary infection occurs with high frequency in a household. The virus can be isolated from the oropharynx and the feces for weeks after infection. There is a seasonal predilection for enterovirus infection, with most cases occurring in the summer and fall. This seasonal pattern coincides with the prevalence of infections caused by the arboviruses, which are mosquito-borne. Eastern and western equine encephalitis virus, La Crosse virus, St. Louis encephalitis virus, and West Nile virus, the newest member of the arboviruses, may cause an aseptic meningitis with symptoms similar to those of the enteroviruses.

All age groups can be infected with enteroviruses; however, young children are most susceptible because they lack the cross-reactive antibodies from repeated exposure to these viruses. Viral meningitis is 5–8 times more common in infants than in adults. Transmission occurs at the time of birth from mother to infant. The maternal disease is usually mild, and a careful history must be taken to detect her illness. Aseptic meningitis in the newborn may mimic bacterial meningitis or herpes simplex meningitis. Distinguishing the etiology of the meningitis is critical since treatment for these infections differs for each.

The majority of enterovirus infections are benign, manifested by fever alone. Other syndromes caused by the enteroviruses include hand, foot, and mouth disease, and painful vesicles on the soft palate and tonsils, with fever, sore throat, and pain on swallowing (herpangina) and painful spasms over the lower ribcage or upper abdomen (pleurodynia). These viruses can also cause life-threatening infections, such as meningitis, myocarditis, encephalitis, neonatal sepsis, and polio. Other than paralytic polio, diseases associated with enterovirus infection, including aseptic meningitis, are not nationally notifiable in the United States. Voluntary participation in the National Enterovirus Surveillance System by state public health labs, private labs, and the CDC enterovirus lab provide the annual statistics. Viruses were recovered most commonly from the CSF (51%) and the stool (17%).

Viruses multiply only in living cells. They lack the necessary synthetic machinery to replicate their genome and viral proteins by themselves. So the virus must "hijack" the host cell to provide energy and relegate its mRNA to produce the necessary viral proteins required for replication. In order for any virus to accomplish this takeover, it must go through several stages (Fig. 17.4). The first stage is the attachment of the virus (virion) to specific cell receptors. The presence or absence of cell receptors determines cell tropism and viral pathogenesis. Enteroviruses have an attachment protein situated in a deep depression ("canyon") around the fivefold axis of the capsid that binds to the host cell. In the second stage the viral particle is engulfed into the host cell within endosomes, an action similar to phagocytosis. In the third stage, called "uncoating," the viral nucleic acid, is separated from the outer structural components. The genome is released as free nucleic acid, and the infectivity of the parent virus is lost. In the fourth stage, viral RNA is translated into polyproteins containing the coat protein and essential replication proteins, and specific mRNA must be transcribed from viral nucleic acid to duplicate the genetic information. In the fifth stage, the new viral particles are assembled into mature virions. In the final stage the new progeny are released and the infected cell lyses. This cytopathic effect (CPE) is observed as the destruction of infected cells.

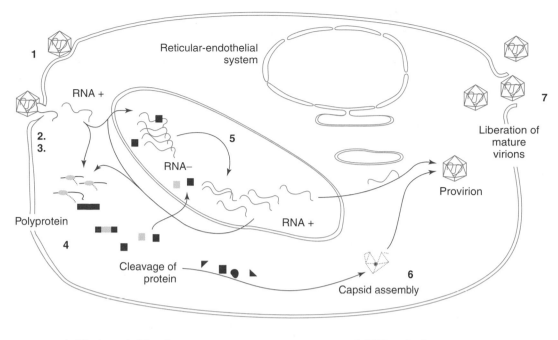

1. Attachment of the virus

2. Penetration of the virus

3. Release of RNA

4. Synthesis of polyprotein

5. RNA replication

6. Capsid added to RNA

7. Mature virion released from host cell

FIGURE 17.4 Replication cycle of an enterovirus.

CPE can be observed in tissue culture when growing these viruses in the laboratory from patient specimens.

Enteroviruses complete the entire replication cycle in 6–10 h. The replication occurs in the epithelial cells and lymphoid tissue of the upper respiratory tract and the gastrointestinal tract. The virus then spreads to other sites, including the CNS, heart, liver, lungs, and skeletal muscle. The target organs vary according to the virus. The lytic nature of the enterovirus leads to cell necrosis and inflammation. The cycle ends with the appearance of circulating neutralization antibodies, interferon, and mononuclear cell infiltration. However, the host immunologic response may backfire to cause further tissue destruction. Antibody to the virus may cross-react with host tissue, resulting in inflammation of the heart (myopericarditis), kidney (nephritis), and muscle tissue (myositis).

17.6. TREATMENT AND PREVENTION

The treatment for most enterovirus infections is supportive. When patients are hospitalized with viral meningitis, antibiotics are administered to cover the possibility of bacterial infection. Acyclovir may be given if there is the possibility of herpes simplex meningitis. However, neither antibiotics nor acyclovir will have any curative effect on an enterovirus infection, and they should be discontinued when the diagnosis of enteroviral meningitis is made. The use of unnecessary antibiotics for enteroviral meningitis has become a more important issue since inappropriate use of antibiotics has lead to the increasing development of bacterial resistance to frequently prescribed antibiotics.

Immunoglobulin therapy has been used prophylactically and therapeutically in the neonate and the immunocompromised host. Immunoglobulin therapy has had some success in patients with agammaglobulinemia and chronic enterovirus infections. The role of immunoglobulin in acute infection remains unproven and is not used in shortlived, non-life-threatening infections.

Molecular characterization of the picornaviruses has led to the development of drugs that target the specific stages of viral replication. Pleconaril is a new antiviral that interferes with the attachment and uncoating of the virus by binding to the viral capsid. It has not been FDA-approved for routine treatment of enterovirus and rhinovirus infections as yet.

17.7. ADDITIONAL POINTS

■ Early in viral meningitis (usually within the first 24 h), PMNs often predominate in the CSF profile. If a patient has a predominance of PMNs in the CSF but a clinical history and exam more suggestive of viral meningitis than bacterial (more indolent presentation), a second LP may be performed 6–12 h after the initial LP to study changes in the CSF profile. The more typical predominance of lymphocytes in the CSF is usually seen at the time of the second LP.

■ Encephalitis is an acute infection of brain parenchyma characterized by fever, headache, and an altered state of consciousness. Focal or multifocal neurological deficits may be present with or without focal or generalized seizure activity. The major causes of encephalitis are herpes simplex types 1 and 2 (HSV-1, HSV-2) and the arthropod-borne viruses. Encephalitis can be differentiated from meningitis on the basis of clinical signs and symptoms and CT or MRI scans demonstrating a hyperintense lesion in the brain.

■ HSV can cause two different syndromes: encephalitis and aseptic meningitis. As a cause of brain infection with or without meningitis (encephalitis), HSV is usually seen in patients without skin lesions. These patients often have a longer clinical course with confusion and disorientation and sometimes seizures. Brain CT or MRI frequently reveals evidence of focal temporal lobe abnormalities.

■ HSV-2 is a cause of aseptic meningitis that may be recurrent. This is most often seen in healthy young patients with primary genital herpes, in which case most patients will have a genital lesion at the time of presentation. Some patients will have recurrent episodes of HSV-2 meningitis with each subsequent outbreak of genital HSV. Rapid diagnosis of herpes simplex CNS disease is critical because it is treatable with the antiviral drug, acyclovir. PCR is considered superior to viral culture of both CSF and brain biopsy with sensitivities of 80–100% and a specificity of 100%.

- Enteroviruses can be present in the stools of people who do not have meningitis. For this reason, just isolating an enterovirus from a specimen other than CSF without CSF confirmation cannot be considered diagnostic for viral meningitis.

- Rapid diagnosis of arbovirus encephalitis can be made by detecting virus-specific IgM in CSF, but this test is available only in reference laboratories. The more common method is by serologic testing using both acute and convalescent sera. One must demonstrate a four-fold or greater rise in titer (from acute to convalescent) to make a serologic diagnosis.

- There has been a decline in the number of vaccine-related poliovirus infections due to the discontinued use of oral (live attenuated) polio vaccine in the United States since 2000.

- Meningitis due to Lyme disease occurs less frequently than does viral meningitis. Differentiating viral meningitis from Lyme meningitis may be difficult since the presence of headache, neck pain, and malaise appears to be a common feature. Patients with Lyme meningitis are more likely to present with swelling of the eyes (papilledema), skin rash (erythema migrans), or cranial neuropathy than are those with viral meningitis. CSF and serum should be tested for antibody to *Borrelia burgdorferi* when there is pertinent epidemiologic and historical data and no viral diagnosis has been confirmed.

- Lymphocytic choriomeningitis (LCM) virus is seen in patients with exposure to the urine or feces of rodents. LCM virus should be suspected in patients with such an exposure history, especially if the CSF glucose is low and the WBC is very high (>1000). Mumps is another viral infection that can cause similar CSF findings. The presence of parotitis or orchitis may be clinical clues to mumps infection.

- The presence of cranial nerve abnormalities should raise your suspicion for carcinomatous or lymphomatous meningitis. A large volume of CSF for cytology should be sent in such cases. Lyme disease, syphilis, and noninfectious etiologies (sarcoid, vasculitis) can also cause cranial neuropathies and CSF pleocytosis.

SUGGESTED READING

CDC, Enterovirus surveillance—United States, 1970–2005, *MMWR* **55**(SS-08):1–20 (2006).

DUBOS, F., B. LAMOTTE, F. BIBI-TRIKI, F. MOULIN, J. RAYMOND, D. GENDREL, G. BREART, and M. CHALUMEAU, Clinical decision rules to distinguish between bacterial and aseptic meningitis, *Arch. Dis. Child.* **91**:647–50 (2006).

KUPILA, L., T. VUORINEN, R. VAINIONPAA, V. HUKKANEN, R. J. MARTTILA, AND P. KOTILAINEN, Etiology of aseptic meningitis and encephalitis in an adult population, *Neurol.* **66**:75–80 (2006).

SAWYER, M. H, Enterovirus infections: Diagnosis and treatment, *Pediatr. Infect. Dis. J.* **18**:1033–1039 (1999).

Neonate with Fever and Vesicular Rash

18.1. PATIENT HISTORY

A 21 year-old woman had a normal spontaneous vaginal delivery of her first baby at 36 weeks of gestation. Although the mother had no pre-natal care, she describes an uncomplicated pregnancy and delivery. The baby weighed 2300 g and had Apgar scores of 8 and 9. The mother had been sexually active in the month up to delivery with a new sexual partner. The baby did well initially, but at four days of age, he was noted to be febrile to 38°C (101.3°F), irritable, disinterested in feeding, and lethargic.

On readmission to the hospital, he was noted to be jaundiced, hypotensive, and have difficulty breathing (dyspneic). On the second hospital day, he developed a scattered vesicular rash on the trunk, extremities, eyes, and mouth. The mother remained asymptomatic, and at her follow-up gynecological evaluation, she had no evidence of uterine infection or genital lesions.

18.2. DIFFERENTIAL DIAGNOSIS

TORCHES is a pneumonic for infections that can be acquired in utero. The pneumonic stands for *t*oxoplasmosis, *o*ther diseases, *r*ubella, *c*ytomegalovirus, *h*erpes simplex, *e*nteroviruses, and *s*yphilis. Other

Medical Microbiology for the New Curriculum: A Case-Based Approach, by Roberta B. Carey, Mindy G. Schuster, and Karin L. McGowan.
Copyright © 2008 John Wiley & Sons, Inc.

diseases include *Listeria monocytogenes*, varicella, human immunodeficiency virus (HIV), and parvovirus.

Because this infant presented initially with the single clinical finding of fever (the rash appeared a day later), he would also have been worked up as a febrile neonate (0–60 days of age). The most common causes of fever (≥38°C or 100.4°F) in neonates include group B streptococcus, *Listeria monocytogenes*, *Streptococcus pneumoniae*, *Staphylococcus aureus*, *Enterococcus* spp., *Escherichia coli*, and other enteric gram-negative rods (*Klebsiella* spp., *Citrobacter* spp., *Enterobacter* spp.). Fever in a neonate can be a sign of arthritis, bacteremia, bacterial or aseptic meningitis, HSV encephalitis, bacterial or viral gastroenteritis, pneumonia, urinary tract infection, or osteomyelitis.

Infectious Causes

The list below represents the combination of organisms acquired in utero plus causes of fever in neonates.

Bacteria

Enterococcus spp.

Escherichia coli and other enteric gram-negative rods (*Klebsiella* spp., *Citrobacter* spp., *Enterobacter* spp.)

Listeria monocytogenes

Staphylococcus aureus

Streptococcus agalactiae [group B streptococcus (GBS)]

Streptococcus pneumoniae

Treponema pallidum (syphilis)

Viruses

Cytomegalovirus (CMV)

Enteroviruses

Herpes simplex virus (HSV)

Human immunodeficiency virus (HIV)

Measles

Parvovirus B19

Rubella

Varicella zoster virus (VZV)

Fungi

Fungi are an unlikely cause of this illness.

Parasites

Plasmodium spp. (extremely rare; to be considered only if mother traveled to or emigrated from an endemic area during pregnancy)

Toxoplasma gondii

CLINICAL CLUES

[?] Skin vesicles and/or seizures in a neonate? Think HSV, and if mother had chickenpox peripartum think VZV. Staphylococcal sepsis can cause pustular skin lesions in the newborn. Syphilis most often causes papulosquamous lesions that involve palms and soles.

[?] Infant less than 7 days of age with fever? Think *L. monocytogenes*, group B streptococcus, *E. coli*, and other enteric gram-negative rods, and rule out meningitis.

[?] Fever in newborn with history of maternal premature rupture of membranes, endometritis, or peripartum wound infection or peritonitis? Worry about β-hemolytic streptococci (groups A and B), *S. aureus*, gram-negative rods, and anaerobes.

[?] Fever and nonspecific symptoms in a newborn? Early-onset meningitis may present without specific CNS symptoms.

18.3. LABORATORY TESTS

A chest x-ray and lumbar puncture (LP) should be performed on this infant because of the presence of fever. During the LP, three or four tubes are obtained for laboratory testing. Refer to Case 16 for collection and transport conditions. A wide variety of laboratory tests should be ordered for the laboratory detection of the pathogens listed in the differential diagnosis. General laboratory tests should include liver function studies, complete blood count and differential, and urinalysis. Blood, urine, and CSF bacterial cultures, as well as CSF Gram stain, should be performed. If the infant has diarrhea, a stool culture for bacterial pathogens should be included. Blood should be obtained for the following serology tests: toxoplasmosis, rubella, and rapid plasma reagin (RPR), a nonspecific screening test for syphilis. In addition, the Venereal Disease Research Laboratory (VDRL) test, a specific test for neurosyphilis, should be performed using CSF.

The diagnosis of viral disease can be enhanced by collecting specimens as early in the disease as possible and by collecting multiple specimens from different body sites. Appropriate specimens from this infant to screen for viral pathogens would include CSF and vesicle scrapings for viral culture; CSF for polymerase chain reaction (PCR), specifically for enterovirus and HSV; skin scrapings for DFA (direct fluorescent antibody) testing for HSV and VZV; and urine for viral culture for CMV. For more extensive discussion on handling of CSF for viral culture, see Case 17.

Specimens for viral testing should be transported to the laboratory as quickly as possible after collection. Specimens should be kept on wet ice or refrigerated, and if transport will take >24 h, specimens should be frozen at –70°C, never at –20°C. Swab and tissue specimens should be placed in a viral transport medium immediately after collection and transported or frozen in that medium. Dacron-, cotton-, or polyester-tipped swabs on plastic or metal shafts are the only acceptable swabs because other types are inhibitory to many viruses. CSF, other sterile body fluids, urine, and stool should be submitted in sterile, leakproof containers and *not* diluted in a viral transport medium. Whole-blood specimens should be collected in an anticoagulant-containing tube, and EDTA (ethylenediaminetetraacetic acid) is the preferred anticoagulant for viral studies requiring white blood cells or plasma for testing.

For viral serology testing, blood should be collected without preservative or anticoagulants (red-topped tube). While a single tube of blood during the acute phase of illness is sufficient to test for IgM antibodies, when testing for virus-specific IgG antibodies, most laboratories will require both an acute specimen and a convalescent specimen taken 10–14 days apart. Specimens collected for nucleic acid testing (RNA or DNA) such as PCR must be handled carefully to avoid destruction of nucleic acid. CSF should be placed on ice immediately after collection and during transport to the laboratory. If transport delay is anticipated, the specimen should be flash-frozen and transported to the laboratory on dry ice.

Because viruses are intracellular organisms, culturing viruses involves inoculating clinical specimens onto a variety of cell lines. A cell line is a monolayer of human or animal cells maintained on the sides of glass or plastic tubes. The cell lines are kept moist and maintained by continuous immersion in a liquid medium containing nutrients. Most laboratories inoculate a battery of different cell lines in order to recover the majority of medically important viruses. A battery used by many labs includes MRC-5 lung fibroblasts (HSV, CMV, adenovirus), Hep-2 cells (adenovirus, HSV), and rhesus monkey kidney cells (enterovirus, adenovirus, influenza, parainfluenza). Once inoculated, cell lines are incubated at 35–37°C for 1–4 weeks depending on the viruses that are suspected. Some viruses such as HSV grow very rapidly (1–3 days); others such as CMV can take much longer (21 days). At least twice a week, the cell lines are inspected microscopically for the presence of virus as indicated by cell death or cell alteration. A change in the cell line due to the presence of virus is called cytopathic effect (CPE), and different viruses have characteristic CPEs.

Shell vial cultures are a modification of conventional cell line cultures. A rounded coverslip containing a monolayer of cells is placed in the bottom of a vial containing growth medium. Specimens are inoculated into the vial, and then the vial is centrifuged. The centrifugation force enhances a virus' ability to infect the cell monolayer, and the result is a more rapid culture. Coverslips with infected cells can then be stained using virus-specific reagents.

The direct fluorescent antibody (DFA) test is a rapid test that is most frequently performed on skin (vesicle) and conjunctival scrapings to screen for HSV and/or VZV. The efficiency of the test depends largely on the collection of a sufficient number of intact infected cells from the lesion. It is best when cells are obtained from the base of an intact vesicle. In general, this test is approximately 70% sensitive when compared with culture for HSV but allows for a rapid diagnosis when positive.

18.4. RESULTS

Bacterial CSF Gram stain and cultures were negative on this baby. DFA tests performed on skin vesicles and conjunctival scrapings were positive

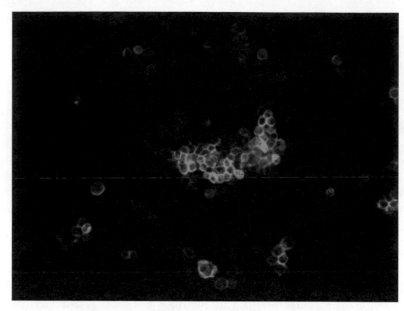

FIGURE 18.1 Positive direct antibody test for HSV.

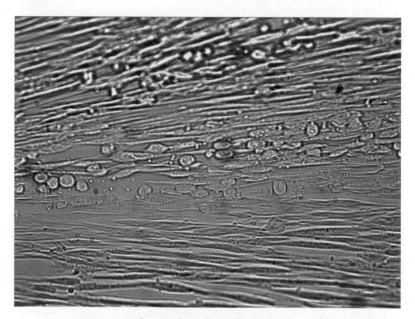

FIGURE 18.2 Cytopathic effect (CPE) seen with HSV.

for HSV and negative for VZV (Fig. 18.1). Viral cultures of CSF and skin vesicle scrapings were both positive for HSV (Fig. 18.2) and CSF PCR was positive for HSV. Because of the speed of the technology, CSF PCR results were available on this patient within 24 h following submittal of the specimen to the laboratory. The sensitivities of HSV PCR assays range within 80–100%, with 100% specificity. Serology tests performed for all other pathogens were negative.

18.5. PATHOGENESIS

Our patient was diagnosed with HSV, which belongs to the family of human herpesvirus that includes herpes simplex types 1 and 2 (HSV-1, HSV-2), varicella zoster virus (VZV), Epstein–Barr virus (EBV), cytomegalovirus (CMV), and human herpesviruses 6, 7, and 8 (HHV-6, HHV-7, HHV-8). They are all DNA viruses that can infect human cells, become latent in the nervous system, and resurrect themselves during times of physical or emotional stress. HSV has a large, double-stranded DNA core surrounded by icosadeltahedral capsid with 62 capsomers (Fig. 18.3). The envelope covering of the virus is sensitive to acids, detergents, solvents and drying. Destruction of the envelope leads to death of the virus.

HSV spreads by close contact, including sexual contact. It enters through the skin or mucosal membranes, replicates, and spreads to the neurons in the infected area. Vesicular lesions filled with virions occur at the site of infection. The virus encodes 11 glycoproteins, which facilitate attachment to the host mucoepithelial cells, fusion with host cell, and production of structural proteins and proteins that allow the virus to escape the immune system. Antibody to the glycoproteins neutralizes extracellular virus. The T helper cells and cytotoxic killer T cells actually destroy the virus. Infections can range from benign in the immunocompetent host to one with a high morbidity and mortality in the immunocompromised patient. The herpesvirus has affinity for neuronal tissue, where it can propagate and remain dormant until it reoccurs following trauma, stress, exposure to sunlight, or fever.

HSV is transmitted person to person, and there are no animal vectors. HSV-1 usually causes fever blisters and cold sores, and most people have

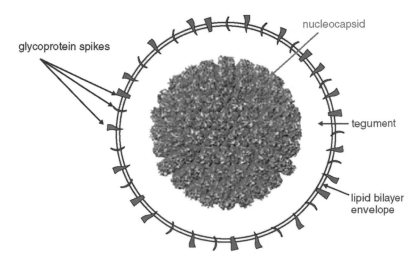

FIGURE 18.3 HSV capsid structure.

antibody to the virus by the time they are adolescents. HSV-2 is more likely to be associated with genital herpes lesions, although genital herpes can be caused by HSV-1 as well. Genital herpes may go unrecognized because it may be asymptomatic. Those with symptoms experience burning and tingling at the site of infection before vesicles emerge. If therapy is given when the early symptoms begin, full-blown disease may be averted.

HSV can be transmitted from infected mother to her infant during the birth process (85%), postpartum (10%), or in utero (5%). Since the newborn lacks cell-mediated immunity, the infection can spread to the liver, lungs, and central nervous system (CNS). Regardless of the time period acquired, one-third of all neonates with HSV disease have CNS disease, resulting in death or mental retardation. Delivery by cesarean section is advised to protect the baby from infection if the mother has active lesions. Transmission is more likely if this is the woman's primary infection with HSV and less likely if this is recurrent disease.

Healthcare workers who examine patients with oral or genital lesions without protective gloves are at risk for infection of the skin on their fingers, called herpetic whitlow. Those who engage in contact sports, such as wrestling, may acquire lesions on their bodies known as *herpes gladiatorum*. Besides the oral and skin lesions described, HSV may cause pharyngitis, stomatitis, eye infection (keratitis), encephalitis, or meningitis.

18.6. TREATMENT AND PREVENTION

For this infant with CNS disease, high-dose acyclovir will be given for 21 days. Treatment for HSV is targeted at destroying the activity of unique enzymes of the virus. The drug acyclovir is given to patients of all age groups to inhibit the activity of DNA polymerase that is essential for viral replication. Acyclovir must be phosphorylated by viral thymidine kinase to activate the drug and stop the elongation of viral DNA.

Resistance to acyclovir occurs from mutations that inactivate thymidine kinase and prevent activation of the drug. A repeat lumbar puncture should be done to determine whether therapy has been successful. A negative PCR for HSV indicates that therapy may be stopped, while a positive HSV PCR indicates that the virus is still replicating and therapy must be continued. For those with only skin, eye, or mouth lesions, treatment is given for 14 days. Suppressive therapy may be administered to pregnant women near the end of pregnancy to decrease shedding of the virus at the time of delivery. Antivirals may reduce the time a person is symptomatic and actively shedding virus. If taken at the first sign of recurrent infection, antivirals may suppress the attack. However, they can never eradicate the virus from the patient.

There is no effective vaccine available at this time to prevent transmission and infection.

18.7. ADDITIONAL POINTS

■ The Apgar test was designed to quickly evaluate a newborn's physical condition immediately after delivery to determine whether they need urgent medical care. The test is usually given to a newborn at 1 min after birth, and then again at 5 min after birth. If there are problems with the baby, an additional score is given at 10 min. The term Apgar, after the American physician Virginia Apgar is frequently used as an the acronym for *a*ctivity, *p*ulse, *g*rimace, *a*ppearance, and *r*espiration. Five factors are used to evaluate the baby's condition, and each factor is scored on a scale of 0–2: activity, pulse (heart rate), grimace response (reflex irritability), appearance (skin coloration), and respiration (rate and effort). The five factors are added together to calculate the Apgar score. Total scores obtainable are between 10 and 0, where 10 is the highest possible score. A score of 7–10 is considered normal, with a score of 4–7 the baby might require some resuscitative measures, and a baby with Apgars of ≤3 requires immediate resuscitation.

■ GBS and *E. coli* produce a polysaccharide capsule that allows the organism to evade phagocytosis by the host cells. Although these organisms differ (one is a gram-positive coccus and the other is a gram-negative rod), both contain sialic acid moieties in their capsules that enable the organisms to penetrate the meninges and cause CNS disease. GBS can cause early-onset disease by infecting the baby in utero or during passage through the birth canal. Late-onset disease occurs days to weeks after birth by contracting the infection from someone who carries the streptococcus on their skin or in their throats. There are several different serotypes of GBS, labeled I, II, III, IV, V, based on the composition of the capsular polysaccharide. Type III is more likely to be associated with meningitis. The American College of Obstetrics and Gynecology, the American Academy of Pediatrics, and the Centers for Disease Control and Prevention (CDC) recommend prenatal screening for vaginal and rectal GBS colonization of all pregnant females at 35–37 weeks' gestation. Intrapartum antimicrobial prophylaxis is given to women who are GBS-positive to prevent invasive disease in their newborns.

■ The strain of *E. coli* that causes neonatal meningitis is *E. coli* K1, named after the capsular antigen that protects the bacteria from phagocytosis. *E. coli* possesses additional virulence factors, fimbriae, which allow the bacteria to bind and attach to the host cell's fibronectin; and lipopolysaccharide (LPS), which elicits an inflammatory response leading to septic shock.

■ *L. monocytogenes* (a gram-positive rod) is acquired by ingestion of the organism in foods contaminated with the bacteria. Soft cheeses, delicatessen meats, and hot dogs have been associated with human infection. Once in the body, *Listeria* attaches and invades the host cells using specialized proteins called "internalins". It becomes a successful intracellular pathogen by forming actin tails that propel the organism through the neighboring cell wall without entering the bloodstream, where it could be attacked by white blood cells or antibodies. When a person eats contaminated food, the organism is carried from the intestine by the lymph or blood to the mesenteric lymph nodes, spleen, and liver. The pregnant woman may experience a flu-like syndrome, but the fetus contracts a more severe infection and may be stillborn.

SUGGESTED READING

CDC, Prevention of perinatal group B streptococcal disease. Revised guidelines from CDC, *MMWR* **51**(RR-11):1–25 (2002).

KIMBERLIN, D. W. Neonatal herpes simplex infection, *Clin. Microbiol. Rev.* **17**:1–13 (2004).

VERGNANO, S., M. SHARLAND, P. KAZEMBE, C. MWANSAMBO, AND P. T. HEATH, Neonatal sepsis: An international perspective, *Arch. Dis. Child. Fetal Neonat. Ed.* **90**:F220–F224 (2005).

VOLANTE, E., S. MORETTI, F. PISANI, AND G. BEVILACQUA. Early diagnosis of bacterial infection in the neonate, *J. Matern. Fetal Neonat. Med.* **16**(Suppl. 2): 13–16 (2004).

Renal Transplant Recipient with Chronic Meningitis

19.1. PATIENT HISTORY

A 46 year-old woman is admitted to the neurological service complaining of left-sided headaches and lethargy for two months. Her past medical history is remarkable for a renal transplant 14 months ago. She has not traveled away from home since her transplant. Her only hobby is gardening in her backyard. On physical exam she appeared lethargic but was easily arousable and in no acute distress. Signs and symptoms of meningeal irritation (meningismus) were not present, and an examination of the vasculature of the eye (funduscopic exam) did not reveal any lesions or papilledema. The oropharynx was clear and review of her cardiovascular and respiratory systems was normal. There was no lymphadenopathy or splenomegaly. Her temperature was 38°C (104°F), pulse 114 beats/min, and blood pressure 150/90 mm Hg. Her neck was supple, but she was not oriented to time or place. Lumbar puncture (LP) revealed clear fluid and an opening pressure of 300 mm H_2O, protein 82 mg/dL, glucose 40 mg%, 44 WBCs/mm^3 (75% lymphocytes), and blood glucose 101 mg%. CSF Gram stain result: moderate WBCs, no organisms seen.

19.2. DIFFERENTIAL DIAGNOSIS

Chronic meningitis is meningitis that lasts for 4 weeks or longer. It is typically insidious in onset and slowly progresses over time. Causes of chronic

Medical Microbiology for the New Curriculum: A Case-Based Approach, by Roberta B. Carey, Mindy G. Schuster, and Karin L. McGowan.
Copyright © 2008 John Wiley & Sons, Inc.

meningitis include infectious agents, malignancy, chronic parameningeal infection, and sarcoid and collagen vascular diseases. Tuberculosis is the leading cause of chronic meningitis and accounts for up to 40% of cases. The epidemiology of infectious chronic meningitis is varied and often linked to geographic and environmental exposures to these pathogens.

Infectious Causes

Infectious causes of chronic meningitis include those listed below.

Bacteria

Actinomyces spp. (associated with oral abscess)

Brucella spp. (associated with unpasteurized dairy products)

Leptospira spp. (exposure to animal urine)

Mycobacteria tuberculosis (especially in the very young or elderly, or in Human Immunodeficiency Virus (HIV) positive)

Mycobacteria other than *M. tuberculosis (MOTT)*

Nocardia spp. (immunodeficiency)

Rare causes: *Listeria monocytogenes, Treponema pallidum, Borrelia burgdorferi*

Fungi

Blastomyces dermatitidis

Candida spp.— seen mostly with intravascular devices

Cryptococcus neoformans

Coccidioides immitis

Histoplasma capsulatum

Sporothrix schenckii

Rare cause: *Aspergillus* spp.

Parasites

Unlikely to cause chronic meningitis.

Viruses

Arbovirus

Cytomegalovirus (CMV)

Echovirus

Flavivirus

Herpes simplex —more commonly an encephalitis rather than meningitis

HIV

Lymphocytic choriomeningitis virus (exposure to rodent urine)

Mumps virus (no vaccination history)

Varicella zoster virus

CLINICAL CLUES

[?] Patient with AIDS? AIDS patients have a lower number of cells in their CSF and, a longer duration of symptoms prior to presentation, and the cell count, protein, and glucose in their CSF may be normal.

[?] Any signs indicating a poor prognosis? Look for a CSF WBC<20 cells/mm^3, CSF cryptococcal antigen >1:1024, and abnormal mental status at presentation.

[?] Patient with chronic meningitis and skin lesions? Skin lesions may be a sign of disseminated fungal infections.

19.3. LABORATORY TESTS

Because the infectious causes of chronic meningitis are so numerous and varied, a careful history and exam are important. It is suggested that one initially concentrate on the most common causes. That would include *M. tuberculosis, C. neoformans*, syphilis, Lyme disease, viruses, and the dimorphic endemic fungal infections. Since TB meningitis often represents reactivation from a previously acquired infection, the patient should be questioned about any prior history of or exposure to TB, even in childhood. A chest x-ray may identify occult pulmonary TB, which may be coexistent with meningeal involvement. Chronic meningitis due to endemic mycoses, such as coccidiomycosis or histoplasmosis, occurs in patients who have lived in endemic areas or traveled there for prolonged periods. Areas endemic for histoplasmosis include Central and South America, and the Ohio and Mississippi River basin area in the United States.

As with acute meningitis, CSF Gram stain plus bacterial, mycobacterial, viral, and fungal cultures are critical tests to perform when making the diagnosis of chronic meningitis. In contrast to acute meningitis, to diagnose both tuberculous and cryptococcal meningitis by culture, large volumes of CSF (10 mL) should be obtained because the number of organisms per milliliter may be very low. With this patient, both the first and fourth tubes of CSF obtained by lumbar puncture should be submitted to the microbiology laboratory. Smears for acid-fast bacteria (AFB) as well as mycobacterial culture should be ordered on the CSF. The sensitivity of CSF AFB smears increases by centrifuging a large volume of CSF to prepare the smear. The laboratory diagnosis of mycobacteria species other than *M. tuberculosis* is dependent on culture. While the purified protein derivative (PPD) skin test for tuberculosis is often negative in cases of TB meningitis, the test should still be performed. Because the agents are initially acquired by inhalation, patients with tuberculous and fungal meningitis may also have evidence of lung disease, and a chest x-ray should be performed. If the x-ray is positive, respiratory specimens (sputum, bronchial lavage, etc.) should also be submitted for bacterial, mycobacterial, fungal, and viral testing. Neurosyphilis, Lyme meningitis, and leptospiral infection are diagnosed by serum and CSF serologic tests. If carcinomatous or lymphomatous meningitis is suspected, a large volume of CSF should be sent for cytology.

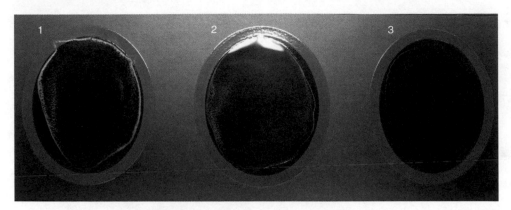

FIGURE 19.1 Latex agglutination test for *Cryptococcus neoformans*.

Other initial laboratory tests should include a WBC count with differential, hemoglobin, hematocrit, and platelet count; serum glucose [which should be taken as close to the time as the lumbar puncture (LP) as possible for comparison with the CSF glucose], blood urea nitrogen (BUN), creatinine, sodium, potassium chloride, carbon dioxide, total protein, albumin, and liver function studies.

The most common test used to make the laboratory diagnosis of *C. neoformans* disease (meningitis or pneumonia) is the cryptococcal latex agglutination test for antigen. This test can be performed on either CSF or serum, but in cases of suspected meningitis, CSF is the specimen to submit for testing. This test detects picogram amounts of the polysaccharide capsule that surrounds the cryptococcal yeast cell. The polysaccharide antigen is shed by the yeast into body fluids. The sensitivity of the test approaches 99%, and antigen detection usually precedes positive CSF cultures for *C. neoformans*. If this test is performed in-house, results may be obtained the same day. When positive, the antigen test result is reported quantitatively as a titer (1:2, 1:4, 1:8, etc.), with higher titers correlating with worsening disease (Fig. 19.1). The titer can also be a prognostic indicator and can be used to monitor therapy.

19.4. LABORATORY RESULTS

Blood cultures: no growth

Mycobacterial, viral, and bacterial CSF cultures: no growth

Mycobacteria sputum cultures × 3: no growth

CSF and sputum AFB smears: negative for acid-fast bacilli

Tests performed for syphilis: from serum [rapid plasma reagin (RPR)] and from CSF [Venereal Disease Research Laboratory (VDRL)] were nonreactive

Lyme serology (ELISA): negative

Leptospirosis serology: negative

Fungal serology testing for dimorphic fungi was not performed

CSF cryptococcal antigen: positive at 1:1024, confirming the diagnosis of cryptococcal meningitis

In general, fungi (yeast and moulds) have longer generation times than do bacteria, and for this reason fungal cultures are maintained for longer periods of time in the lab than are bacterial cultures. While many yeasts are capable of growing within 48 h, some moulds can take as long as 3–4 weeks of incubation to grow. Most fungal cultures are held and examined for a total of four weeks before completion. As with bacterial cultures, a battery of different media are inoculated, which will support the growth of various fungi. CSF submitted for fungal culture is centrifuged, and then the sediment is plated onto a variety of fungal media, some of which contain antibiotics. In contrast to the prokaryotic bacteria, fungi are eukaryotic organisms whose cell walls contain chitin and/or cellulose. Fungi are usually grouped according to their morphological appearance as either a yeast or a mould. Yeasts are unicellular organisms, generally round to oval-shaped, which reproduce by budding (Fig. 19.2). They can appear as single, circular, creamy, sometimes mucoid, or sometimes pigmented colonies when grown on solid agar plates (Fig. 19.3). Since colonies of many yeast species may appear similar on routine culture media, a chromogenic agar may be used to demonstrate the presence of more than one species in a culture (Fig. 19.4). Like bacteria, yeasts are frequently identified using microscopic morphology and biochemical tests. In contrast, moulds are multicellular filamentous organisms, which are composed of thread-like filaments called hyphae that when woven together form a structure called

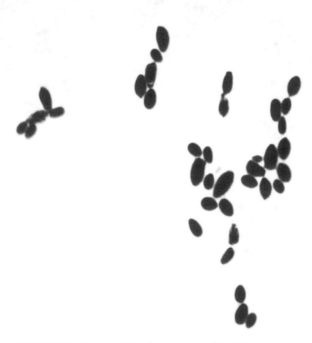

FIGURE 19.2 Gram stain showing oval budding yeasts.

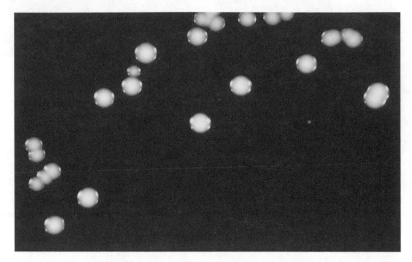

FIGURE 19.3 Colonies of yeast on blood agar.

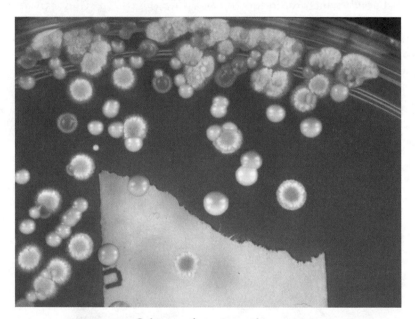

FIGURE 19.4 Colonies of yeasts on chromogenic agar.

a mycelium. Moulds are usually identified by their macroscopic (Fig. 19.5) and microscopic morphologies and growth at different temperatures. For identification to species, moulds frequently must be induced to produce asexual spores (Fig. 19.6).

In contrast to bacterial cultures incubated at 35–37°C, all fungal culture media should be incubated at 30°C under aerobic conditions and held for four weeks.

After 3 days of incubation, mucoid nonpigmented colonies typical for *C. neoformans* were observed on Sabouraud agar and 5% sheep blood agar

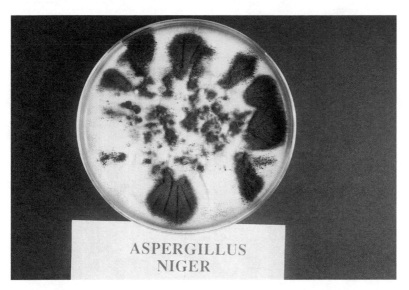

FIGURE 19.5 Macroscopic view of a mould on Sabouraud's agar.

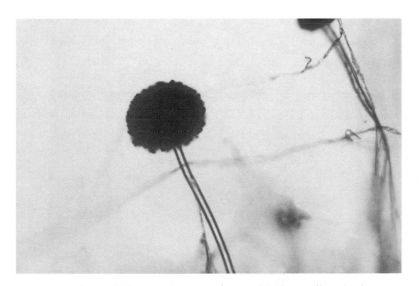

FIGURE 19.6 Microscopic view of a mould (*Aspergillus niger*).

plates (Fig. 19.7). The organism was identified as *C. neoformans* using a rapid urease test (Fig. 19.8) and phenol oxidase disk test, both of which are positive for *C. neoformans* (30 min–4 h).

19.5. PATHOGENESIS

C. neoformans is an opportunistic pathogen causing disease in immunocompromised patients, especially those with T-lymphocyte deficiencies

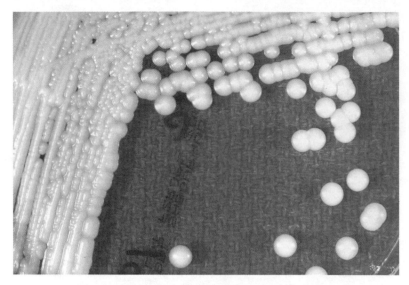

FIGURE 19.7 Mucoid colonies of *Cryptococcus neoformans*.

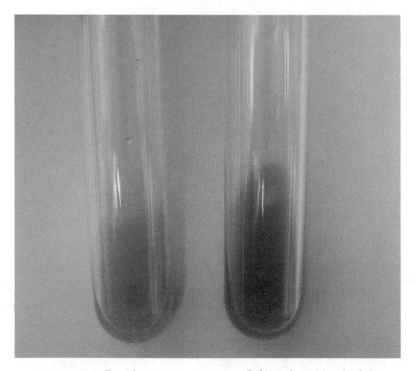

FIGURE 19.8 Rapid urea tests: negative (left) and positive (right).

and those on high-dose corticosteroid therapy. This yeast is an important cause of meningitis for patients with uncontrolled or advanced HIV infection, Hodgkin's disease, systemic lupus erythematosus, lymphocytic leukemia, and solid organ transplant. However, infections can occur in an immunocompetent host who is exposed to a large inoculum of the yeast.

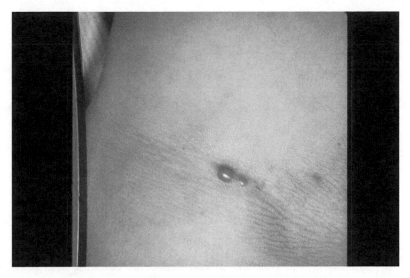

FIGURE 19.9 Skin lesion from *Cryptococcus neoformans.*

The lung is usually the primary site of infection since the organism is acquired by inhalation. Once it invades the body, the organism has a high predilection to spread to the brain and meninges. There are two varieties and four serotypes of *C. neoformans* based on the capsular polysaccharide antigen: serotypes A and D (var. *neoformans*) and serotypes B and C (var. *gatti*). Serotypes A and D are found in the excreta of pigeons, chickens, and Canadian geese. The organisms survive in desiccated alkaline soil, so our patient probably inhaled the organism while gardening. Person-to-person spread of infection has not been documented.

Because of our patient's T-cell suppression induced by the antirejection drugs given post-transplant, the organisms disseminated from her lungs by a hematogenous route to her meninges. Once in the brain, the organisms may become an expanding intracerebral mass causing focal neurologic deficits. CNS disease may be associated with other evidence of disseminated infection, such as skin lesions, as observed on the forearm of our patient (Figs. 19.9, 19.10).

The polysaccharide capsule of *C. neoformans* has antiphagocytic activity and is a major virulence determinant for this yeast. Strains lacking the thick mucoid capsule are more easily phagocytized and are less virulent in animal models. The capsule can be visualized in histological sections when material is stained with mucicarmine (Fig. 19.11). In a wet mount of CSF mixed with India ink, the capsule can be seen as a negatively stained area around the yeast cell (Fig. 19.12). On repeated subculture of the organisms on artificial media, the yeast cell loses its capsule.

The production of phenol oxidase is another virulence factor for *C. neoformans*. This enzyme catalyzes the conversion of phenolic compounds, such as dopamine, present in high concentration in the CSF, to melanin. Melanin accumulates in the cell wall and may protect the organism from host immune cells. Mutants lacking this enzyme are avirulent in animal models and more easily phagocytized.

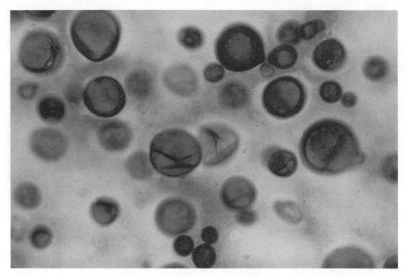

FIGURE 19.10 Skin touch prep positive for *Cryptococcus neoformans* (PAS stain).

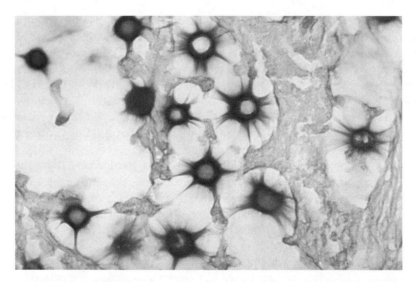

FIGURE 19.11 Mucicarmine stain of capsule of *Cryptococcus neoformans*.

19.6. TREATMENT AND PREVENTION

Untreated cryptococcal meningoencephalitis is uniformly fatal. A combination of amphotericin B and 5-flucytosine (5-FC) was used to treat our patient with cryptococcal meningitis. A two-drug regimen is standard therapy since the combination therapy will clear infection from the CSF more quickly and with less toxicity than will a single drug alone. In patients with underlying HIV infection, the CSF cannot be permanently cleared of the cryptococcal organisms, and so these patients are given chronic suppression therapy (fluconazole) for life to prevent relapse. Patients without

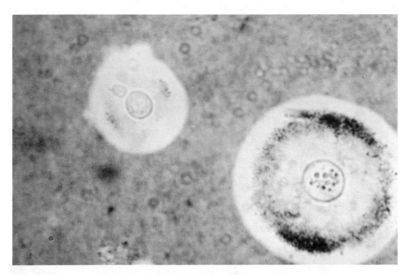

FIGURE 19.12 India ink prep showing large capsule of *Cryptococcus neoformans*.

HIV do not require suppression therapy after the initial treatment for meningitis.

Most patients without AIDS respond to two weeks of combination therapy, at which time oral fluconazole may be given to replace the amphotericin and 5-FC. The duration of treatment with fluconazole varies from three to six months. Immunosuppressed patients, such as solid organ transplant recipients, require more prolonged courses of therapy. If a patient does not improve after two weeks of combination therapy, a repeat LP should be performed, and both drugs continued until the cultures are negative. The opening pressure of the CSF on LP should be monitored closely. Patients with initially high opening pressures are at greater risk for adverse neurological events. Similarly, acute neurologic deterioration during treatment may indicate elevated intracranial pressure, which can be treated with removal of CSF or a surgically placed shunt for decompression, if necessary.

Serial antigen titers can be used to monitor response to therapy. Three months after treatment, our patient's cryptococcal antigen titer in the CSF had decreased to 1:2 and her symptoms had resolved. Patients whose posttreatment CSF antigen remains >1:8 have a higher likelihood of relapse.

19.7. ADDITIONAL POINTS

- Serum from patients with invasive infections from the yeast *Trichosporon beigelii* and the bacteria *Capnocytophaga canimorsus* and *Stomatococcus mucilaginosis* will give false-positive results with the cryptococcal antigen latex test due to cross reacting polysaccharides.

- Prior to availability of the cryptococcal antigen latex test, colloidal carbon solutions such as India ink were used in an attempt to microscopically visualize encapsulated organisms such as *Cryptococcus*. Because large numbers of yeast cells were necessary for the test to be positive,

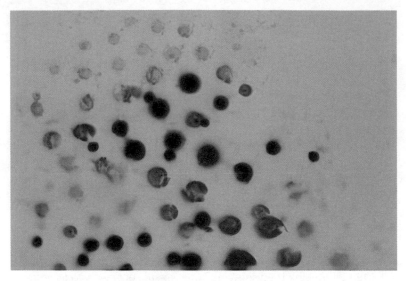

FIGURE 19.13 Gram stain of *Cryptococcus neoformans*.

it was negative in many cases of true meningitis and considered an unreliable and insensitive test. Most laboratories no longer perform India ink preparations with CSF (Fig. 19.12).

■ While considered an insensitive method of detection, on occasion *Cryptococcus* spp. can be seen on a Gram stain smear of centrifuged CSF. The yeast cells stain weakly and will appear gram-negative or have some gram-positive stippling (Fig. 19.13).

■ An enzyme immunoassay (EIA) is also available for the detection of cryptococcal polysaccharide antigen. The test is thought to be more sensitive than latex assays, but because it is more expensive, it requires an instrument for reading and interpretation of results, and results in a longer turnaround time, and thus is not offered in most laboratories.

■ HIV patients with CD4 counts <100 have a higher likelihood of developing cryptococcal meningoencephalitis.

SUGGESTED READING

BICANIC, T. AND T.S. HARRISON, Cryptococcal meningitis, *Br. Med. Bull.* **72**:99–118 (2005).

COHEN, B. A., Chronic meningitis, *Curr. Neurol. Neurosci. Rep.* **5**:429–439 (2005).

PAPPAS, P. G., Therapy of cryptococcal meningitis in non-HIV-infected patients, *Curr. Infect. Dis. Rep.* **3**: 365–370 (2001).

SAAG, M. S., J. R. GRAYBILL, R. A. LARSEN, ET AL., Practice guidelines for the management of cryptococcal disease, *Clin. Infect. Dis.* **30**:710–718 (2000).

Man with Acute Fever and Periumbilical Pain

20.1. PATIENT HISTORY

A 25 year-old male presented to the emergency department complaining of severe abdominal pain. The pain was steady, unrelenting, and aggravated by any motion. For the past week he had loss of appetite and intermittent nausea, vomiting, and fever and thought he had the "stomach flu." Two days ago, he developed some pain around the umbilicus, which then shifted to the right lower abdomen. Today he awoke with acute, diffuse belly pain and tenderness. His temperature was 39°C (102.2°F), heart rate 110 beats/min, blood pressure 110/68 mm Hg, and respirations 20 breaths/min. His abdomen was distended. No bowel sounds were appreciated, and his abdomen was markedly tender to minimal palpation. There was tensing of abdominal muscles (guarding) and pain on releasing pressure on the abdomen (rebound tenderness). Laboratory studies revealed an elevated WBC count of 14.6 /mm^3 with 89% polymorphonuclear neutrophils. An x-ray of the abdomen showed a paralytic ileus with free air visible under the diaphragm. He was scheduled for emergency surgery.

20.2. DIFFERENTIAL DIAGNOSIS

This patient presented with signs and symptoms of peritonitis, a localized or general inflammation of the membrane lining the abdominopelvic wall

Medical Microbiology for the New Curriculum: A Case-Based Approach, by Roberta B. Carey, Mindy G. Schuster, and Karin L. McGowan.
Copyright © 2008 John Wiley & Sons, Inc.

(peritoneum). The finding of free air under the diaphragm points to per-foration of the GI tract. When mucosal epithelial cells are traumatized or perforated, normal flora organisms spill into sterile cavities and tissues. Abdominal trauma or a ruptured appendix frequently leads to peritonitis after normal gastrointestinal (GI) flora enters into the abdominal cavity. In females a tubo-ovarian abscess may present with similar signs and symptoms. GI flora of the large bowel is predominantly anaerobic bacteria (90%), enteric gram-negative rods, enterococci, yeasts, streptococci, and staphylococci.

Infectious Causes

Organisms that are frequent causes of bacterial appendicitis or peritonitis include those listed below.

Bacteria

Anaerobes:

> *Bacteroides* spp.—gram negative rods that account for 10–12% of human fecal flora
>
> *Clostridium* spp.—gram-positive rods, with spores
>
> *Fusobacterium* spp.—gram-negative rods, some with pointed (fusiform) ends
>
> *Peptostreptococcus* spp.—gram-positive cocci

Gram-negative rods:

> *Campylobacter* spp.
>
> *Enterobacter* spp.
>
> *Escherichia coli*
>
> *Klebsiella* spp.
>
> *Salmonella* spp.
>
> *Shigella* spp.

Gram-positive cocci:

> *Enterococcus* spp.
>
> *Staphylococcus* spp.
>
> *Streptococcus* spp.

Fungi

> *Candida* species are normal GI flora and could be part of a polymicro-bial infection following ruptured appendix.

Parasites

> Parasites are not normal GI flora; *Echinococcus* cyst is rare.

Viruses

> Viruses are not normal GI flora; viruses are not a cause of peritonitis.

Non-infectious Causes

Diverticulitis

Duodenal ulcer

Foreign body

Gastrointestinal malignancy

Inflammatory bowel disease

Pancreatitis

CLINICAL CLUES

? Presence of fever and leukocytosis with abdominal pain? Patients with high fever and elevated WBC should be suspected of having a perforated appendix.

? Localized pain in the lower right quadrant? Patients with appendicitis often have initial abdominal pain in the periumbilical area that localizes to the right lower quadrant.

? Localized left-sided pain? Patients with diverticulitis most often have left-sided abdominal pain.

? Absent or diminished bowel sounds and rebound tenderness? Symptoms indicate peritonitis. Patients with appendicitis and other causes of peritonitis may have pain on rectal or vaginal exam.

20.3. LABORATORY TESTS

Laboratory testing of aspirated peritoneal fluid can provide immediate information, particularly if attempting to distinguish between intraperitoneal infection and hemorrhage. If present, fluid should be submitted for Gram stain plus aerobic and anaerobic bacterial culture. The centrifuged fluid should also be examined for WBCs, RBCs, and amylase. If fever is present, blood cultures should be performed using a two-bottle set that includes an aerobic bottle and an anaerobic bottle. A WBC count with differential, liver function tests, and a serum amylase test should also be ordered.

A Gram stain should always be performed on specimens submitted for anaerobic culture. Many anaerobic bacteria have a characteristic morphology on Gram stain, and this can provide valuable information to clinicians early in the course of illness when it can affect the choice of antibiotics. Awareness of the presence of possible anaerobes frequently expands antibiotic coverage for a patient. Morphologically, *Bacteroides fragilis* appears as a pale, unevenly staining gram-negative rod with rounded ends and bipolar staining (Fig. 20.1). In comparison, *Fusobacterium* spp. stain gram-negative with pointed rather than rounded ends (Fig. 20.2). *Clostridium* spp. appear as large, broad, or thin gram-positive rods, with or without spores (Fig. 20.3). Peptostreptococci appear as gram-positive cocci in chains, but compared with enterococci or streptococci, *Peptostreptococcus*

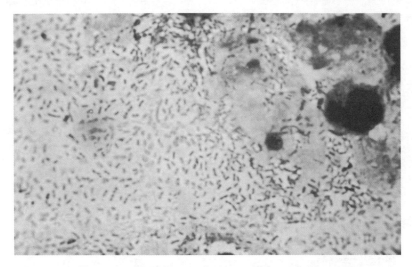

FIGURE 20.1 Short gram-negative rods compatible with *Bacteroides* species.

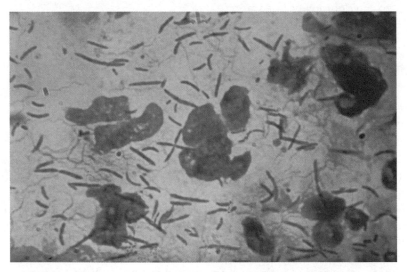

FIGURE 20.2 Long gram-negative rods with pointed ends compatible with *Fusobacterium* species.

spp. are generally smaller in size. Because anaerobic cultures can take much longer to process, clues obtained from Gram stain can be critical. When bacteria observed on Gram stain are not recovered by subsequent aerobic culture, the presence of anaerobes should always be suspected.

Anaerobes are bacteria that cannot grow in the presence of oxygen. Those that cannot tolerate any levels of oxygen are called "strict" or obligate anaerobes. Those that can tolerate and grow in reduced amounts of oxygen are called microaerophilic. Clinical specimens submitted for anaerobic culture require special handling for organisms to be recovered successfully. More than with other fastidious bacteria, careful attention is

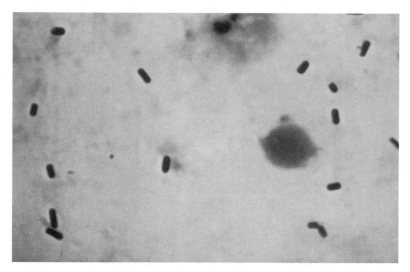

FIGURE 20.3 Large rectangular gram-positive rods compatible with *Clostridium* species.

needed to be paid in the collection and transport of specimens potentially containing anaerobes. Some specimen types are unacceptable for anaerobic culture such as sputum, throat swabs, superficial wounds, feces, urine, and cervical or vaginal specimens because of the presence of normal anaerobic flora. Specimens that would be appropriate for anaerobic culture would include normally sterile body fluids, abscess contents, deep-wound aspirates, tissue or biopsy samples, transtracheal aspirates, and suprapubic urine aspirates.

The presence of normal anaerobic flora on most human mucous membranes means that these areas need to be avoided when obtaining specimens for anaerobic culture. Specimens submitted on swabs are inadequate and in some labs unacceptable, and efforts should be made to submit fluid or tissue samples. Specimens should be placed into an oxygen-free tube or vial for transport to the laboratory (Fig. 20.4). Tissue biopsy specimens can also be placed into oxygen-free tubes or vials. Many of these vials contain a small amount of buffered transport medium, which enhances the viability of both strictly anaerobic and facultatively anaerobic bacteria. Specimens submitted for anaerobic culture need to be transported to the laboratory as quickly as possible (≤ 2 h).

Once anaerobic specimens are received in the laboratory, initial processing involves the use of media specifically designed to recover anaerobes. After inoculation, the medium is incubated in special jars, pouches, anaerobic chambers, or glove boxes to maintain an anaerobic environment (Fig. 20.5) and incubated at 35–37°C. Many laboratories do not initially examine anaerobic culture media until they have incubated for a minimum of 48 h. Identification of anaerobes requires the use of biochemical tests in a similar fashion as that used with aerobes, as well as more complicated methodologies such as gas–liquid chromatography. Under well-defined conditions, anaerobes will produce characteristic metabolic

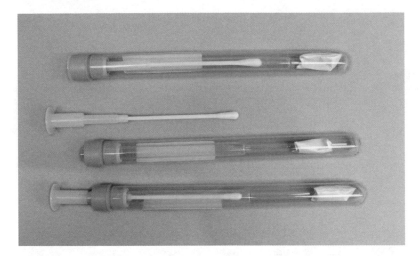

FIGURE 20.4 Anaerobic transport system.

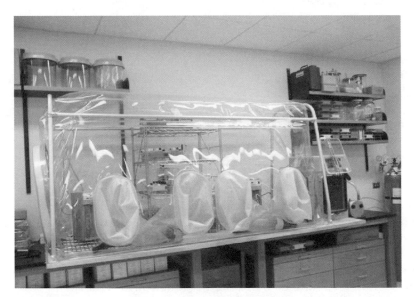

FIGURE 20.5 Anaerobic chamber.

by-products. Because many anaerobes require prolonged periods of incubation for growth, anaerobic cultures are time-consuming and a final result should not be expected for 4–6 days after submission to the lab.

20.4. RESULTS

The Gram stain of the patient's peritoneal fluid revealed many WBCs, many gram-negative rods, many gram-positive non spore-forming rods, and few gram-positive cocci in short chains. Cultures later grew *B. fragilis* group, *Clostridium perfringens, E. coli*, and *Enterococcus* spp.

General laboratory characteristics of clinically significant anaerobes are as follows:

Bacteroides. Members of this genus are normal flora inhabitants of the mouth and upper respiratory tract, GI tract, and urogenital tract of humans and animals. Eleven species of this genus are in the *B. fragilis* group and are the major constituents of the lower GI tract and therefore are always encountered in intra-abdominal infections. As a group they are considered the most virulent of the *Bacteroides* and are universally β-lactamase-positive. Most species can be identified on the basis of colony morphology, pigment production, fluorescence under UV light, rapid and traditional biochemical tests, and gas–liquid chromatography.

Clostridium. Members of this genus are normal flora inhabitants of the lower GI tract of both humans and animals. In addition, a number of species (*C. tetani, C. botulinum*) are soil and environmental inhabitants and are not part of normal human flora. Because of this epidemiologic difference, clostridial infections can be acquired by trauma or ingestion of contaminated food as well as through endogenous mechanisms. Members of this genus are identified in the laboratory using a wide variety of methods, including appearance on a variety of specialized media, biochemical tests, and gas–liquid chromatography. Most *Clostridium* species are highly sensitive to penicillin; however, production of β-lactamase has recently been documented in this group, and isolates should be tested.

Fusobacterium. Members of this genus are normal flora inhabitants of the mouth and upper respiratory tract, lower large intestine, and vaginal tract. While there are presently 12 species of *Fusobacterium*, *F. nucleatum,* and *F. necrophorum* are the species most commonly isolated from humans. The fusobacteria differ morphologically on Gram stain from the *Bacteroides* in that they are fusiform gram negative rods with pointed ends. This genus is differentiated from *Bacteroides* spp. in the laboratory by their ability to fluoresce under UV light, their susceptibility to kanamycin, and their ability to produce unique metabolic by-products. Members of this genus are capable of producing β-lactamase and should be tested.

Peptostreptococcus. Members of this genus are normal flora of the mouth and upper respiratory tract, GI tract, and urogenital tract. They are most often found in mixed infections along with anaerobic gram-negative rods and microaerophilic streptococci. The anaerobic cocci grow well on most types of nonselective anaerobic media within 48–72 h. Peptostreptococci are sensitive to penicillin since they do not produce β-lactamase.

Susceptibility testing of anaerobes is not routinely performed at most hospitals, but many hospitals document patterns of resistance for their region by testing isolates every few years. All laboratories should be capable of performing a rapid test for detection of β-lactamase enzymes, which should be performed routinely on all anaerobic gram-negative and gram-positive rods.

20.5. PATHOGENESIS

Three main factors in anaerobic infections contribute to the clinical syndrome: (1) the patient's endogeneous flora content from the GI tract, GU tract, or oropharyngeal mucosa causes the infection; (2) there is an alteration of the host's tissues by trauma, loss of oxygenated blood supply (hypoxia), or neoplasm, to create the proper anaerobic environment; and (3) anaerobic infections are polymicrobial and usually mixed with aerobic gram-negative bacteria, which reduce the oxygen in the environment and provide the complex nutrients required by anaerobic microorganisms.

Few anaerobic pathogens are primary invaders of healthy epithelium, except for *F. nucleatum*, a slender gram-negative rod found in the oral mucosa that causes a severe infection in the tonsils and pharynx, leading to a potentially fatal disease, known as Ludwig's angina.

Various virulence factors are shared by most anaerobes. Metabolic by-products, such as volatile fatty acids, sulfur compounds, and amines, lead to tissue damage and cause the foul-smelling odor associated with anaerobic infections. Hydrolytic enzymes and proteases dissolve tissue components, allowing the anaerobes to spread and procure necessary nutrients. The lipopolysaccharide of anaerobic gram-negative rods has less endotoxin activity than do enteric gram-negative rods, but it reduces the opsonic activity of serum and stimulates gingival inflammation when it is present in the oral cavity.

The most commonly isolated anaerobic bacteria in human infections are listed in the Table 20.1.

20.6. TREATMENT AND PREVENTION

Because of the time-consuming laboratory methods used to isolate and identify anaerobes, antibiotic treatment for this group of bacteria is frequently empiric. Our patient has signs and symptoms of peritonitis due to perforation of the gastrointestinal tract with spillage of bacterial flora into the peritoneal cavity. The clinical presentation is most consistent with an appendix that perforated. The combination of surgical drainage and antibiotics is essential. Antibiotics used alone are not likely to be effective. This is also true when treating cases of gas gangrene. Once the majority of the pus is removed, the appropriate choice of antibiotics is dictated by the site of the infection. Abscesses "below the belt" require antimicrobial agents that will be effective in the face of β-lactamases that destroy penicillins and first-generation cephalosporins, such as cefazolin. With anaerobes, the main mechanism of antibiotic resistance is the production of β-lactamase enzymes. An antibiotic that combines a β-lactam plus a β-lactamase inhibitor (ampicillin/sulbactam or ticarcillin/clavulanic acid) or a second-generation cephalosporin (cefoxitin) is active against *Bacteroides*

TABLE 20.1.	Virulence Factors of Anaerobic Bacteria and the Mechanism of Action	
Anaerobic Bacteria	Virulence Factor	Activity
Bacteroides fragilis	Capsular polysaccharide	Antiphagocytic, inhibits complement activity
	Lipopolysaccharide	Reduces opsonic activity of complement
	Superoxide dismutase	Allows organism to survive in oxygen
	Fimbriae (pili)	Adherence to host epithelial cells
Clostridium botulinum	Neurotoxins A–F	Acts on CNS, inhibiting the release of acetylcholine at cholinergic synapses, leading to irreversible paralysis
Clostridium difficile	Toxin A	Enterotoxin causing diarrhea
	Toxin B	Cytotoxin causing roundup of cells, observed in tissue culture
Clostridium perfringens	α-Toxin (Phospholipase C)	Destroys cell membrane and lyses erythrocytes, causing gas gangrene
	β-Toxin	Produces necrotic enteritis (pig-bel syndrome)
	ε-Toxin	Increases permeability of gut wall to absorb more toxin, leading to systemic lethal effects
	Enterotoxin	Causes food poisoning 8–24 h after eating
Clostridium tetani	Tetanospasmin	Binds to gangliosides in the CNS, suppresses inhibitory neurotransmitters, causing muscle spasm
Fusobacterium nucleatum	Lectins	Adherence to host cells
	Lipases	Damage host cell membrane
	Hemolysins	Damage host tissue

species that are usually β-lactamase-positive as well as the enteric gram-negative rods.

Other acceptable choices of antimicrobial therapy include clindamycin and metronidazole that have activity against anaerobes, but they must be combined with other antibiotics that are effective against enteric gram-negative rods.

Penicillin G can be given to treat anaerobic infections that are "above the belt," such as dental abscesses, lung, and brain abscesses, which are caused by a combination of anaerobes, such as *Fusobacterium* species, and microaerophilic streptococci. Similarly, penicillin can be used to treat infections with *C. perfringens*. Other *Clostridium* species, however, may be resistant to broad-spectrum penicillins and second- and third-generation cephalosporins.

Antibiotics that are not indicated for anaerobic infections include the aminoglycosides (gentamicin, tobramycin, and amikacin), which are almost totally ineffective against anaerobes. Likewise, most fluoro-quinolones are not recommended for treatment of mixed infections involving anaerobes since they have low activity against these organisms.

Our patient was treated successfully with a combination of piperacillin/tazobactam to cover his infection caused by anaerobes and enteric gram-negative rods. The patient underwent exploratory laparotomy, where a perforated appendix with pus in the peritoneal cavity was noted. A washout of the peritoneal cavity was performed, with appendectomy. The incision was left open to heal by secondary intention.

20.7. ADDITIONAL POINTS

- Botulism is a classic anaerobic disease and is seen in three different forms: foodborne botulism, infant botulism, and wound botulism. Foodborne botulism results from the ingestion of food containing preformed toxin of *Clostridium botulinum*. It is most frequently associated with faulty home canning, particularly of vegetables. Spores of *C. botulinum* normally found in dirt and soil are not sufficiently killed by heating during the canning process, and then organisms multiply during storage and produce potent neurotoxins, which are ingested. Foodborne botulism has also been associated with canned saltwater or freshwater fish.

- Infant botulism, also called "floppy baby syndrome," is a result of infants ingesting spores of *C. botulinum*, which then go on to produce neurotoxins in vivo. Infants ingest the spores when they consume honey, corn syrup, and other food products. Clinically the infants are lethargic, are hypotonic, and have muscle weakness and loss of head control. For this reason they appear floppy.

- Wound botulism is a rare illness and is a complication of traumatic wound infections where the wound site contains *C. botulinum* organisms. From the effects of the neurotoxin being produced at the wound site, patients present with symmetrical descending weakness or paralysis.

- The laboratory diagnosis of botulism is made by demonstrating the presence of botulinum toxin. For infant botulism, appropriate specimens are stool and serum; for wound botulism, stool, serum, and tissue are appropriate samples. Testing for botulinum toxin and culturing for *C. botulinum* from clinical specimens is performed by state public health laboratories and the Centers for Disease Control and Prevention.

- The disease tetanus is caused by *Clostridium tetani* and is characterized by difficulty in swallowing, muscle rigidity, difficulty opening the mouth (trismus or lockjaw), and muscle spasms in a patient with a previous or present wound infection. The symptoms are the direct result of exotoxin produced by *C. tetani* located at a wound site. Tetanus is a clinical diagnosis; confirmatory laboratory tests are not routinely available. Because treatment involves early recognition and treatment with antitoxin, recovery of organism is not essential in making the diagnosis. On Gram stain, the organism has the appearance of tennis rackets because of the terminal location of the spore (Fig. 20.6). Tetanus is preventable through the use of immunization with tetanus toxoid and appropriate wound care.

- *Clostridium perfringens* is known for causing two diseases: gas gangrene and food poisoning. *C. perfringens* food poisoning is caused by the

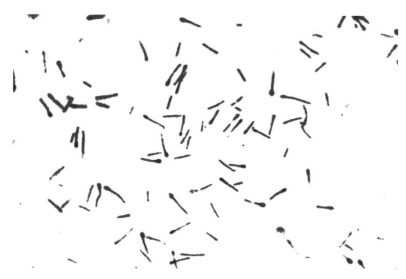

FIGURE 20.6 Gram-positive rods with terminal spores compatible with *Clostridium tetani.*

ingestion of food containing vegetative cells of enterotoxin-producing *C. perfringens*. After ingestion, the vegetative cells multiply and sporulate, releasing the enterotoxin in vivo. The illness is characterized by diarrhea and abdominal cramping, with no fever. Symptoms typically occur 7–15 h after ingesting food contaminated with high concentrations of the organism, and the illness typically lasts no longer than 24 h. Because *C. perfringens* can be present in small numbers in human fecal flora and raw food samples, laboratory confirmation of this disease requires the detection of high levels of *C. perfringens* in the food and patient feces plus the demonstration of enterotoxin in patient feces. This testing is performed only by state public health laboratories and the Centers for Disease Control and Prevention.

■ Gas gangrene caused by *C. perfringens* is a fulminant infection that, without treatment, rapidly progresses to shock and death. It develops in severe traumatic open wounds when there is muscle damage and contamination with dirt or material containing spores of the organism. The disease has been seen most often as a result of war wounds where severe trauma, gross soil contamination, and delayed medical or surgical intervention are most common, but it can also be seen following other types of traumatic wounds (gunshot, crush injuries, motor vehicle accidents, colon and biliary tract surgeries). Clinical manifestations include brown or bronze skin discoloration, foul- or sweet-smelling serosanguinous discharge, cutaneous bullae, crepitance, and edema. Pain is commonly out of proportion to physical findings, and the progression to shock and toxemia can be rapid. Radiologic findings show subcutaneous gas, a hallmark of the disease, which is a direct result of damaged muscle carbohydrate fermentation by *C. perfringens*. Current therapy for *C. perfringens* gas gangrene involves aggressive surgical debridement, antibiotic treatment, and use of hyperbaric oxygen therapy.

■ *Clostridium difficile* is one of the most common anaerobic infections seen in humans, but, unlike other *Clostridium* spp., *C. difficile* is not associated with abscesses or wounds. *C. difficile* is the etiologic agent of antibiotic-associated colitis and pseudomembranous colitis and is thought to account for 25% of all antibiotic-associated diarrhea. This is the only anaerobic infection that can be passed from person to person, and thus *C. difficile* is the most infectious cause of nosocomial diarrhea in adults in the United States. The bacterium produces two toxins: toxin A, an enterotoxin; and toxin B, a cytotoxin. Diagnosis of *C. difficile*–induced disease is usually made by testing for the presence of toxins A and B in stool, a test routinely performed in most hospital laboratories.

■ *Prevotella* and *Porphyromonas* spp. are anaerobic gram-negative rods and gram-negative coccobacilli similar to *Bacteroides* spp. that are frequently seen in polymicrobic infections. They are identified by their ability to fluoresce brick red when exposed to ultraviolet light, or their production of brown or black pigment.

SUGGESTED READING

DUERDEN, B. I., Virulence factors in anaerobes, *Clin. Infect. Dis.* **18**(Suppl 4):S245–S320 (1994).

HATHEWAY, C. L., Toxigenic clostridia, *Clin. Microbiol. Rev.* **3**:66–98 (1990).

STEVENS, D. L. ET AL., Practice guidelines for the diagnosis and management of skin and soft tissue infections, *Clin. Infect. Dis.* **41**:1373–1406 (2005).

Man with Two Weeks of Fever and a Systolic Murmur

21.1. PATIENT HISTORY

A 64 year-old male was brought to a local tertiary-care hospital with a 2-week history of shortness of breath, fever, chills, and rigor. Of note, two months prior to admission he had extensive dental work performed but felt fine in the weeks following the procedure. On examination he was a frail, quite ill-appearing man in moderate discomfort with deep rapid respiration. His blood pressure was 94/54 mm Hg, pulse rate 100 beats/min, and respiratory rate 30 breaths/min, and he had a fever of 39°C (102.2°F). There was no lymphadenopathy. His teeth were in good repair, and his eyes had no hemorrhages or exudates. Chest exam revealed few basilar rales, and a systolic cardiac murmur was detected at the cardiac apex with radiation to the axilla. Abdomen was nontender and liver and spleen not palpable. Multiple nonpalpable erythematous bluish-red lesions were noted on his toes (Fig. 21.1), and a splinter hemorrhage was also seen under the nail of his right index finger. Transthoracic echocardiography showed a severely altered posterior leaflet of the mitral valve with a large (3 × 3 mm) vegetation. Initial laboratory results included a WBC count of 14,000 [50% polymorphonuclear neutrophils (PMNs), 10% bands, 40% lymphocytes], hematocrit 42%, urinanalysis 2+ protein, 10–20 RBC, 5–10 WBC; and an erythrocyte sedimentation rate of 67 mm/h. Chest x-ray showed a widened mediastinum and clear lung fields.

Medical Microbiology for the New Curriculum: A Case-Based Approach, by Roberta B. Carey, Mindy G. Schuster, and Karin L. McGowan.

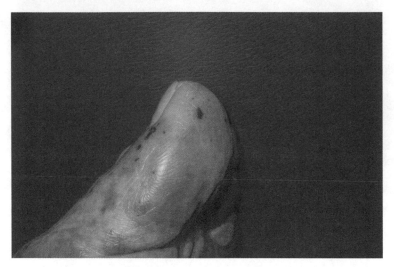

FIGURE 21.1 Janeway lesion.

21.2. DIFFERENTIAL DIAGNOSIS

This patient's clinical findings are compatible with the diagnosis of infective endocarditis (IE), which is an infection of the heart's inner lining (endocardium) or the heart valves. The two major types of IE are acute and subacute, based on the tempo and severity of the clinical presentation. Acute IE usually involves normal valves and is a rapidly progressive illness. Subacute IE usually involves only abnormal valves, and symptoms can be present for weeks or even months before patients present.

Conditions associated with an increased risk of IE include structural abnormalities due to congenital heart disease, valvular heart disease, rheumatic fever, prior heart valve surgery, prior IE, or an artificial (prosthetic) heart valve. Poor dental hygiene or recent dental surgery, long-term hemodialysis, injection drug use, long-term indwelling intravenous catheters, chronic renal disease, diabetes mellitus, systemic lupus erythematosus, and surgery involving respiratory, intestinal, or genitourinary tract mucosa are also additional risk factors.

Infectious Causes

The bacterial pathogens causing IE consist largely of organisms that are normal skin and oral flora, as well as fastidious organisms, and the HACEK group of organisms. Other infectious agents include those listed below.

Bacteria

Corynebacterium spp.

Enterococcus spp.

Fastidious organisms:

Bartonella spp., especially B. quintana

Brucella spp.

Chlamydia psittaci

Coxiella burnetti

Legionella spp.

Gram-negative enteric rods

Haemophilus spp.

Neisseria gonorrhoeae

HACEK (acronym derived from first letters of genuses) organisms:

    Haemophilus aphrophilus

    Actinobacillus (*Haemophilus*) *actinomycetemcomitans*

    Cardiobacterium hominis

    Eikenella corrodens

    Kingella kingae

Mycobacterium spp.

Nocardia spp.

Pseudomonas aeruginosa and other *Pseudomonas* spp.

Staphylococcus aureus

Staphylococcus spp.—coagulase-negative

Streptococcus spp.—groups A, B, C, and G

Streptococcus pneumoniae

Streptococcus, viridans group:

    S. anginosus

    S. bovis

    S. mitis

    S. mutans

    S. salivarius

Streptococcus-like, formerly nutritionally variant strep

    Abiotrophia spp.

    Granulicatella spp.

Fungi

Aspergillus spp.

Candida spp.

Histoplasma capsulatum

Other yeasts and moulds, accounting for <10%

Viruses

Viruses are not a cause of infective endocarditis.

Parasites

Parasites are not a cause of infective endocarditis.

TABLE 21.1.	Risk Factors for Acquiring Fastidious or Unusual Pathogens Causing Endocarditis
Risk Factor	Organism
Farm animal exposure or unpasteurized milk	*Coxiella burnetti, Chlamydia psittaci, Brucella* spp.
Dog or cat exposure	*Pasteurella* spp., *Capnocytophaga* spp.
Intravenous drug use	*Corynebacterium* spp., fungi, polymicrobial IE
Homeless persons, alcoholism, HIV	*Bartonella* spp.
Immunocompromised host	*Corynebacterium* spp., *Listeria* spp., *Legionella* spp.
Solid organ transplant	*Aspergillus fumigatus, Candida* spp.
Poor dental hygiene, recent dental surgery	HACEK group, nutritionally variant streptococci
Gastrointestinal lesions	*Clostridium septicum, Streptococcus bovis*
Travel to endemic areas	*Histoplasma capsulatum, Coxiella burnetti, Brucella* spp.

Noninfectious Causes

Atrial myxoma

Cardiac neoplasms

Thrombotic nonbacterial endocarditis (also known as marantic endocarditis)

Risk Factors

Epidemiologic clues are helpful indicators when unusual or fastidious organisms should be considered (Table 21.1).

CLINICAL CLUES

[?] Hemorrhagic lesions in nailbeds, eyes, or extremities? Think infectious endocarditis.

[?] Fever and fatigue following recent dental manipulation or poor dentition? Think infectious endocarditis with an organism from the oral cavity.

[?] Fever and fatigue following GI or GU manipulation? Think infectious endocarditis with gram-negative rods or enterococci.

[?] Vague symptoms such as depression, low back pain, fatigue, and weight loss? Think endocarditis. Many patients do not have fever or leukocytosis and present with nonspecific symptoms.

21.3. LABORATORY TESTS

The gold standard test for making the laboratory diagnosis of IE is documentation of a continuous bacteremia (>30 min in duration) based on blood culture results. To diagnose subacute IE, three to six separate sets of blood cultures (aerobic and anaerobic) taken over a 2-day period will detect 92–98% of cases in patients who have not received antibiotics. For acute IE, three sets of blood cultures drawn at 30-min intervals (from separate venipunctures) will detect 99% of cases. Blood cultures should be obtained prior to initiation of empiric antibiotics. A 1:10 blood-to-broth ratio is critical to maximize blood culture results. A minimum of 10 mL of blood should be obtained for each culture (adults) (Fig 21.2). Fastidious organisms may require special culture media, special incubation conditions, or prolonged incubation, and the laboratory should be alerted when fastidious organisms are suspected. If initial blood cultures fail to yield an infectious agent after 48 h incubation, additional blood cultures should be taken, assuming that the patient is not receiving antibiotics. Prior use of antibiotics is the most common cause of false-negative blood cultures when attempting to make the diagnosis of IE. Other causes are fastidious organisms and testing inadequate volumes of blood. Serologic tests can be used to diagnose several fastidious organisms, namely, *Coxiella burnetti*, *Chlamydia* spp., *Brucella* spp., and *Legionella* spp.

The microbiology laboratory should be notified if fastidious or unusual organisms (*Legionella, Mycobacteria, Bartonella*) are suspected because special culture techniques or requirements may be necessary to recover these organisms. Transthoracic echocardiogram is usually performed, and transesophageal echocardiogram may be done to better visualize the valves and look for myocardial abscess formation. Electrocardiograms should be done periodically to detect conduction abnormalities, which may be

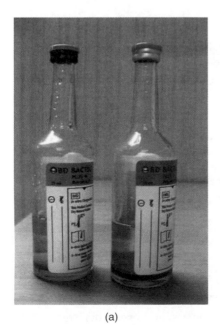
(a)

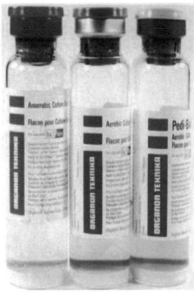
(b)

FIGURE 21.2 Blood culture bottles.

TABLE 21.2.	Other Laboratory Tests that May Support the Diagnosis of Infective Endocarditis
Test	Observation
Erythrocyte sedimentation rate (ESR)	Elevated in most IE patients
Rheumatoid factor (RF)	Elevated in 50% of IE patients
Serum creatinine	Frequently elevated in IE
Serum complement levels	Decreased with IE
Peripheral leukocyte count	Normal or moderately elevated
Platelet count	Documented thrombocytopenia
RBC count	Mild to moderate normocytic–normochromic anemia common
Urinalysis	Proteinuria and microscopic hematuria common

associated with erosion of the infection into the myocardial conduction system.

A number of nonspecific tests are often used to support the diagnosis of IE, but none are considered a definitive way to make the diagnosis (Table 21.2).

In the event of culture negative IE, if surgery is part of the treatment regimen, then removed heart valves and/or vegetations can be Gram-stained, cultured, and histopathologically stained to aid in the choice of antibiotics and length of treatment. Special histopathologic stains can be used for identifying fungi (Grocott–Gomori methenamine silver) (Fig. 21.3), mycobacteria (Ziehl–Neelsen, auramine–rhodamine) (Fig. 21.4), *Bartonella* spp. (Warthin–Starry, Giemsa, and Gram) (Fig. 21.5), and *Coxiella* and *Legionella* spp. (Gimenez).

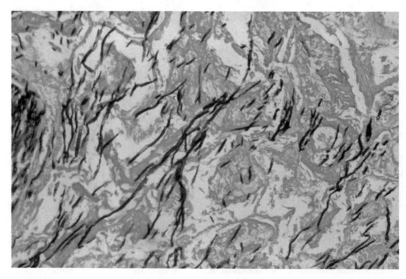

FIGURE 21.3 Grocott–Gomori methenamine stain showing hyphae in tissue.

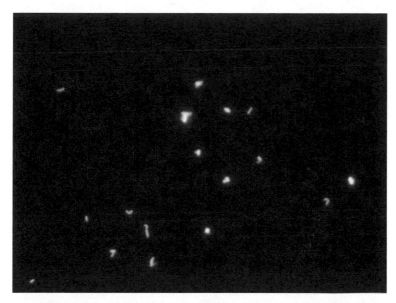

FIGURE 21.4 Auramine–rhodamine fluorochrome stain.

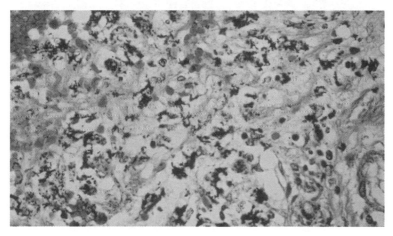

FIGURE 21.5 Warthin–Starry stain.

Six sets of blood cultures were drawn from the case patient over the course of two days. Each set included an anaerobic bottle and an aerobic bottle, each inoculated with 10 mL of blood.

21.4. RESULTS

After 24 h incubation, five of six sets of blood cultures yielded gram-positive cocci in chains (Fig. 21.6). The bacteria grew on sheep blood agar and chocolate agar at 35°C in 5% CO_2 and appeared as tiny α-hemolytic, gray colonies (Fig. 21.7). The colonies were catalase-negative, optochin (P disk)–resistant, leucine aminopeptidase (LAP)–positive, and pyrrolidonyl arylamidase (PYR)–negative, and failed to grow in the presence of

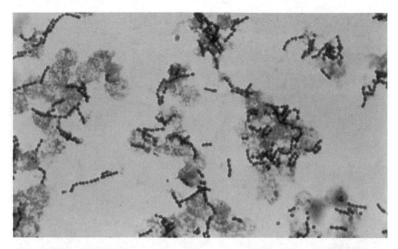

FIGURE 21.6 Gram-positive cocci in pairs and chains compatible with streptococci.

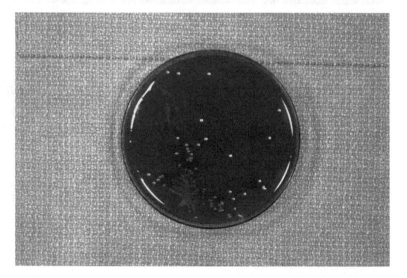

FIGURE 21.7 α-Hemolytic colonies of *Streptococcus mitis* on blood agar.

bile esculin and 6.5% NaCl. The organism was identified as a viridans streptococcus, and further biochemical testing identified it as *Streptococcus mitis*.

The term viridans streptococci is used to describe a group of α-hemolytic or nonhemolytic streptococci that are normal inhabitants of the human respiratory tract, female genital tract, and gastrointestinal tract. Most viridans streptococci do not possess a specific cell wall group antigen (Lancefield groups A, B, C, etc.). Viridans streptococci are capable of causing a variety of serious infections, most notably endocarditis. The clinical significance of viridans streptococci and their response to antibiotics can differ between species, so it is important to identify them to the species level. Viridans streptococci can be divided into five major groups:

1. *S. mutans* group, the major cause of dental caries
2. *S. bovis* group

3. *S. salivarius* group

4. *S. mitis* group

5. *S. anginosus/S. milleri* group, associated with abscess formation

Antimicrobial susceptibility testing on the *S. mitis* isolated from our case patient showed intermediate activity to penicillin (MIC = 1 μg/mL), and susceptibility to ceftriaxone, cefepime, clindamycin, erythromycin, and vancomycin.

21.5. PATHOGENESIS

Unlike *S. pyogenes* (group A strep), the viridans streptococci lack a library of virulence factors that allow them to prey on a healthy host. The viridans streptococci require a break in the natural protective barriers to gain entry into the bloodstream of the host. Trauma to the mucosa, immunosuppression, or insertion of a medical device allows these opportunistic pathogens to breach the skin or mucous membranes and cause serious infections.

Abnormalities of the heart valve create irregular surfaces where sterile platelet–fibrin deposits accumulate at sites where blood flows. Circulating bacteria may stick and colonize these areas, and the host responds with the deposition of fibrin, platelets, and white cells. As the host response increases, a friable vegetation is created that results in an abnormal opening and closing of the heart valve, and a murmur is heard on auscultation. Infectious endocarditis is detected by positive blood cultures and radiographic changes. The aortic and mitral valves are the most commonly infected. On the right side of the heart, the tricuspid valve is more commonly infected in IV drug users. Vegetations may break off from the valve and embolize microorganisms to other organs, such as the kidneys, brain, or myocardium, and these are known as septic emboli. Glomerulonephritis may occur from the deposition of antigen–antibody and complement in the renal glomeruli, which causes hematuria, proteinuria, or renal failure.

Infective endocarditis has been classified into acute or subacute forms with different clinical presentations. Acute endocarditis is a destructive, rapidly progressing infection of a normal heart valve by a virulent microorganism, such as *S. aureus*. Subacute endocarditis is a slower, insidious infection of heart valves that have been previously damaged, allowing organisms lacking virulence factors to infect the tissue. Endocarditis of native heart valves is most often caused by viridans streptococci or other commensals of the oral cavity. Prosthetic valve endocarditis is commonly caused by coagulase-negative staphylococci.

21.6. TREATMENT AND PREVENTION

Treatment for infective endocarditis is based on the pathogen recovered. Because many different microorganisms can cause this infection, every effort is made to recover a pathogen from the blood or heart valve tissue. If left untreated or treated inappropriately, the disease is ultimately fatal. Antimicrobial therapy must be administered for 4–6 weeks because the organisms are embedded deeply in the fibrin matrix and are slowly dividing. It is difficult for antibiotics and host white cells to penetrate the tissue and reach their target, which also dictates the need for prolonged therapy. For many organisms, two antimicrobial agents are given in combination to ensure synergistic killing activity, commonly a cell wall active antibiotic, such as penicillin plus an aminoglycoside. Our patient was given penicillin and gentamicin. The addition of gentamicin for the first two weeks of therapy will increase the rate of killing of the streptococci and avoid relapse. If our patient had been allergic to penicillins, a cephalosporin or vancomycin would be substituted as the cell wall active antibiotic depending on the severity of the allergy. Surgery to replace the damaged heart valves may be indicated if heart failure occurs, if the bloodstream does not become sterile with antibiotics alone, if multiple embolic complications occur, or if a myocardial abscess is present. Additionally, some organisms that cause endocarditis, such as fungi, almost always require valve replacement for cure.

Because the patient will receive long-term therapy with potentially toxic drugs, serum is tested at intervals to monitor the level of gentamicin or vancomycin. Since gentamicin may damage the kidneys (nephrotoxic) and impair hearing (ototoxic), baseline hearing levels are obtained at the start of therapy and monitored during the course.

Patients with a known risk for endocarditis due to prior damage to their heart valve are advised to take prophylaxis when they undergo dental manipulation (cleaning) or undergo certain medical procedures. Usually a single antibiotic, such as penicillin or ampicillin, is administered orally just prior to the procedure to eradicate transient bacteremia that occurs during the procedure. Prophylaxis should be discontinued promptly after the procedure to avoid extended exposure to antibiotics that would increase the occurrence of antibiotic-resistant microorganisms.

21.7. ADDITIONAL POINTS

- A number of skin lesions are associated with IE. These include petechiae on the skin, conjunctivae, palate, and under fingernails (called "splinter hemorrhages"), Janeway lesions, and Osler nodes. Janeway lesions are painless hemorrhagic lesions of long-term duration that occur on the palms of the hands (Fig. 21.1) and soles of the feet. The underlying mechanism is thought to be due to circulating immune complexes of antigen, antibody, and complement. Osler nodes are small painful red–purple nodules located primarily in the pads of the fingers and toes. They represent microemboli to small vessels and microabscesses (Fig. 21.8).

- Other clinical findings associated with IE that can be observed during physical exam include Roth spots (white-centered hemorrhagic lesions on the retina); conjunctival hemorrhage; joint pain; enlarged spleen; enlargement and clubbing of the fingers; swelling of feet, legs, and abdomen; and a new heart murmur or a change in a previous murmur. Embolic events may present with major neurological symptoms, such as stroke, headache, visual impairment, convulsions, intracranial bleeds, mycotic aneurysm, and mononeuritis.

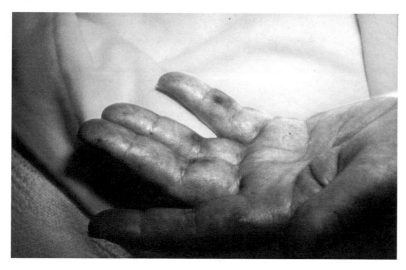

FIGURE 21.8 Osler's node.

■ Although the viridans streptococci lack virulence factors to make them aggressive pathogens, one cannot assume that they are universally susceptible to antimicrobial agents. They carry genes that alter their penicillin-binding proteins so that cell wall active antibiotics may not be effective when used alone. It is important that susceptibility testing be performed on viridans streptococci causing IE so that the most active antimicrobial agent can be selected for therapy.

■ Approximately 5% of cases of suspected IE yield negative blood culture results and are termed culture-negative IE. Polymerase chain reaction (PCR)–based tests have been used to diagnose infective endocarditis due to *Tropheryma whipplei* and *Bartonella* spp. and may be a promising tool for establishing a microbiological diagnosis in patients with culture-negative IE.

SUGGESTED READING

American College of Cardiology/American Heart Association 2006 guidelines for the management of patients with valvular heart disease, *Circulation* **114**: e84–e231 (2006).

BADDOUR, L. M., W. R. WILSON, A. S. BAYER ET AL., Infective endocarditis: Diagnosis, antimicrobial therapy, and management of complications, *Circulation* **111**: 3167–3184 (2005).

BASHORE, T. M., C. CABELL, AND V. FOWLER, JR., Update on infective endocarditis, *Curr. Probl. Cardiol.* **31**: 274–352 (2006).

BROUQUI, P. AND D. RAOULT, Endocarditis due to rare and fastidious bacteria, *Clin. Microbiol. Rev.* **14**: 177–207 (2001).

SEXTON, D. J. AND D. SPELMAN, Current best practices and guidelines. Assessment and management of complications in infective endocarditis, *Infect. Dis. Clin. N. Am.* **2**: 507–521 (2002).

QUAGLIARELLO, V., Infective endocarditis: Global, regional, and future perspectives, *JAMA* **293**: 3061–3062 (2005).

Young Man with Fatigue and an Abnormal Liver Test

22.1. PATIENT HISTORY

During a routine pre-employment medical exam, a 24 year-old unmarried man was found to have abnormal liver test results. When questioned further, he admitted to fatigue and vague abdominal pain that had persisted for the past 5 weeks. He denied ever receiving a blood transfusion or using injection (IV) drugs. He did admit to unprotected sexual encounters with multiple partners while in college. As a college graduation present, he vacationed 5 months ago in Trinidad and reports that he received several tattoos during the trip. His physical exam was within normal limits. A rectal exam revealed yellow-brown stool and a negative stool guaiac for occult blood. The abnormal lab tests included an elevated alanine aminotransferase (ALT) of 175 International Units per liter (IU/L) (normal = 5–60 IU/L) and an elevated aspartate aminotransferase (AST) of 145 IU/L (normal = 5–43 IU/L). Bilirubin and alkaline phosphatase levels were both normal. The company physician then advised him to see his own primary-care physician.

22.2. DIFFERENTIAL DIAGNOSIS

This patient reported two significant risk factors during his physical exam: participating in unprotected sex with multiple partners and getting tattoos

Medical Microbiology for the New Curriculum: A Case-Based Approach, by Roberta B. Carey, Mindy G. Schuster, and Karin L. McGowan.
Copyright © 2008 John Wiley & Sons, Inc.

while vacationing outside the United States. Despite his denial of using intravenous drugs, he was still potentially exposed to unclean, unsterilized needles while being tattooed. Tattooing and body piercing pose health risks because both processes expose the needles to blood and body fluids. As a result, a person who undergoes either procedure risks getting an infection that is carried through blood. This would include hepatitis B, hepatitis C, tetanus (caused by *Clostridium tetani*), and human immunodeficiency virus (HIV). ALT and AST are transaminase enzymes that are produced in the liver. The liver uses transaminase enzymes to metabolize amino acids and form proteins. Many different factors can cause ALT and AST enzymes to increase, including infections. The word hepatitis means inflammation of the liver, without indicating a specific cause.

Infectious Causes

Organisms that could cause hepatitis include those listed below.

Bacteria

Bartonella henselae

Borrelia burgdorferi (Lyme disease)

Brucella melitensis

Coxiella burnetii (Q fever)

Legionella pneumophila

Leptospira interrogans

Mycoplasma pneumoniae

Rickettsia rickettsii

Salmonella typhi

Treponema pallidum

Viruses

Adenovirus

Cytomegalovirus

Enterovirus

Epstein–Barr virus (which causes infectious mononucleosis)

Flavivirus—cause of dengue fever

Hepatitis viruses A, B, C, D, E (the most common causes of viral hepatitis in the United States are A, B, and C)

Herpes simplex virus

Human immunodeficiency virus (HIV)

Rubella

Varicella zoster virus

Yellow fever virus

Fungi

Aspergillus spp. (in people with compromised immune systems)

Blastomyces dermatitidis

Candida spp. (in people with compromised immune systems)

Coccidioides immitis

Cryptococcus neoformans

Histoplasma capsulatum

Penicillium marneffei

Parasites

Ascaris lumbricoides

Clonorchis sinensis

Echinococcus granulosus

Entamoeba histolytica

Fasciola hepatica

Leishmania donovani

Plasmodium spp.

Schistosoma spp.

Strongyloides stercoralis

Toxocara canis

Toxoplasma gondii

Noninfectious Causes

Autoimmune hepatitis

Excessive alcohol intake or alcoholic liver disease

Exposure to toxic chemicals or poisons

Fatty liver (fat buildup in liver cells: steatohepatitis)

Inherited liver diseases

Liver tumors

Medications and certain herbs

CLINICAL CLUES

[?] Complaints of dark-colored urine and light-colored stools? Evidence of yellow discoloration of the skin (jaundice) or yellow discoloration of the sclera (scleral icteris)? Think viral hepatitis.

[?] History of recent tattoos or other body piercing and abdominal pain? Think hepatitis B or C.

[?] Fatigue and jaundice following travel out of the country? Think hepatitis A.

[?] History of needlestick in a healthcare worker? Think hepatitis B or C.

> **?** Severe or fulminant hepatitis? Think coinfection of hepatitis B and D, which is often more severe.
>
> **?** Evidence of a serum sickness–like illness with rash, fever, and arthritis? Think hepatitis B.

22.3. LABORATORY TESTS

When originally seen, this patient had abnormal AST and ALT levels but normal bilirubin and alkaline phosphatase levels. While he was fatigued and had vague abdominal pain, other hallmark findings on physical exam such as jaundice, scleral icterus, dark urine, diarrhea, rash, hepatomegaly, and splenomegaly were absent in this patient. His history of unprotected sex with multiple partners and tattooing place him at risk for hepatitis B virus (HBV), hepatitis C virus (HCV), and HIV, and he should be tested for these using serology tests. In addition, a complete battery of liver function tests (LFTs) should be performed. This would include measuring albumin, bilirubin, cholesterol, total protein, and various liver enzymes [ALT, AST, and γ-glutamyltranspeptidase (GGT)]. A complete blood count to check for anemia and blood cell abnormalities as well as prothrombin time (PT) and partial thromboplastin time (PTT) studies and a complete urinanalysis should also be performed. An abdominal x-ray can show changes in liver size, the presence of liver abscesses, abnormal mineralization, and circulatory abnormalities. Depending on the results of initial testing, abdominal ultrasound of the liver, biliary tree, and spleen may need to be performed.

The laboratory diagnosis of HBV and HCV is achieved through the use of serology tests detecting antibodies or antigens. The primary test used to detect HCV antibody is an enzyme immunoassay, which detects IgG antibody to HCV. The test is performed using serum, it is highly sensitive and specific (99%), and a negative test result is adequate to exclude the diagnosis of HCV in immunocompetent patients. A positive result is an indicator of recent or past infection. False-negative HCV antibody results can occur due to a 1–6-week window period that occurs between the onset of symptoms and antibody production. A HCV RNA PCR test is recommended to detect HCV infection in seronegative individuals who are immunocompromised and to discriminate chronic from acute infection in patients who have previously tested positive for HCV antibody. In addition, the HCV RNA PCR test can be quantitative, and this provides useful information about prognosis, transmission, and response to therapy.

To understand HBV serology, you must be familiar with a number of definitions related to HBV serology testing (see Table 22.1). There are several tests used to detect the presence of HBV antibodies and others to detect HBV antigens. Serology testing for HBV is usually ordered as a hepatitis B panel as shown in Table 22.1.

A graph of the acute serologic response to HBV is shown in Fig. 22.1, and the chronic serologic response is shown in Fig. 22.2.

To diagnose acute hepatitis, IgM HBcAb, HBsAg, anti-HBsAg, and anti-HCV are ordered as a panel to detect recent infection with HBV or HCV. In hepatitis B infection, during the incubation period (1–6 months),

TABLE 22.1.	Use and Interpretation of Serologic Markers for the Diagnosis of Hepatitis B	

Serologic Indicator	Abbreviation	Use/Interpretation
Hepatitis B surface antigen	HBsAg	HBsAg in serum indicates acute or chronic infection. During acute disease, this antigen appears before onset of symptoms and before elevation of ALT. The presence of this antigen indicates infectivity. In those with chronic HBV infection, this test remains positive.
Hepatitis B surface antibody	anti-HBs or HBsAb	HBsAb is a protective antibody that neutralizes HBV. It usually appears during early convalescence and after low levels or no levels of HBsAg are detectable. This antibody persists for life and indicates recovery, when the virus is no longer present and the patient is not infectious. It is also the *only* antibody detected in people who have received the HBV vaccine.
Total hepatitis B core antibody (includes IgM and IgG)	anti-HBc or HBcAb	Total HBcAb (IgM + IgG) indicates exposure to the virus and viral replication. HBcAb appears shortly (1–4 weeks) after HBsAg during acute disease and then persists for life; thus its presence indicates acute or chronic infection. HBcAb is not a good marker for acute disease.
IgM antibody to hepatitis B core antigen	IgM anti-HBc or IgM HBcAb	This antibody appears during acute or recent HBV infection and persists for ~6–12 months. On occasion, it can persist at low levels during chronic infection.
Hepatitis B e-antigen	HBeAg	This antigen is a marker of active disease and high infectivity. Persistence for ≥ 8 weeks after acute disease indicates progression to a chronic carrier state. HBeAg levels are monitored to determine the effectiveness of treatment. When treatment is successful, HBeAg disappears and antibodies against this antigen appear.
Hepatitis B e-antibody	anti-HBe or HBeAb	This antibody is produced in response to HBeAg and will be present in those who have recovered from acute HBV. In chronic HBV disease, HBeAb becomes positive when the virus is eliminated from the body or goes into hiding.

HBSAg appears 2–7 weeks prior to symptoms and usually clears during convalescence (unless infection becomes chronic). Antibody to HBsAg (HBsAb) usually becomes detectable as HBsAg clears. Sometimes, there is a "window period" where HBsAg has cleared but HBsAb is not yet detectable. IgM HBcAb may be helpful in diagnosing acute hepatitis B in this setting. In patients with chronic (duration >6 months) hepatitis, or with elevated ALT or AST, HBsAg, total HBcAb, and anti-HCV are ordered.

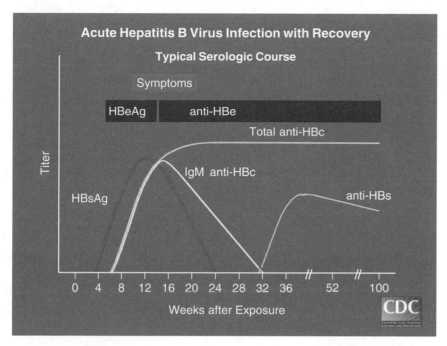

FIGURE 22.1 Acute serologic response to hepatis B virus.

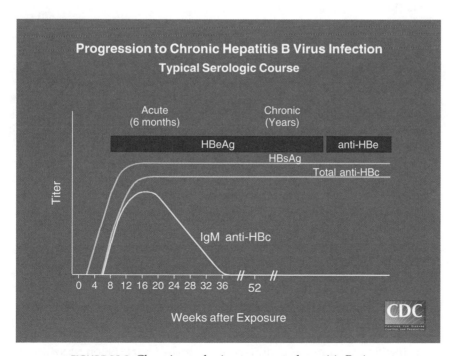

FIGURE 22.2 Chronic serologic response to hepatitis B virus.

A hepatitis B DNA quantitative PCR test (HBV DNA) is a more sensitive test than HBeAg for detecting virus in the bloodstream (viremia) and viral infectivity. Although not performed in all laboratories, when available, it is used in conjunction with regular serologic tests. It is an early predictor of disease progression and is also used to monitor the effectiveness of treatment, particularly in those with chronic HBV infections. It is not used to diagnose acute infection.

22.4. RESULTS

The following laboratory results were obtained on this patient:

ALT: 100 IU/L

AST: 75 IU/L

Bilirubin: normal

Alkaline phosphatase: normal

Albumin: normal

Total protein: normal

Globulin: normal

CBC: normal

Prothrombin: normal

Partial thromboplastin time: normal

HBsAg: negative

HBsAb: positive

IgM HBcAb: positive

Anti-HCV: negative

The HBV serology results indicate immunity due to a natural infection from HBV, and this patient is no longer infective. With the exception of his elevated ALT and AST results, which have decreased since his pre-employment physical, all other liver function studies and coagulation markers are normal, and these results correlate with the HBV serology results.

22.5. PATHOGENESIS

Our patient has hepatitis B (also known as serum hepatitis), which is one of a group of viruses known to attack the liver and cause icteric changes, such as jaundice, and an increase in liver enzymes. Although many viruses may damage the liver and cause hepatitis, the most common causes of viral hepatitis are known by alphabet letters: A, B, C, D, E, and G. Each hepatitis virus has its own unique characteristics, and they all belong to different viral families. Hepatitis A virus (HAV, also known as infectious hepatitis) and E virus are similar in their clinical presentation, and both are acquired

TABLE 22.2. Comparison of Biologic and Clinical Characteristics of Hepatitis Viruses

	Hepatitis A	Hepatitis B	Hepatitis C	Hepatitis D	Hepatitis E
Type of virus	Picornavirus	Hepadnavirus	Flavivirus	Deltavirus	Calicivirus
Nucleic acid	RNA	DNA	RNA	RNA	RNA
Transmission	Fecal/oral Sexual — —	Blood Body fluids Sexual Perinatal	Blood Perinatal — —	Blood Body fluids Sexual Perinatal	Fecal/oral — — —
Incubation (days)	15–50	28–160	14–160	15–64	15–45
Chronic disease/carrier	No	Yes	Yes	Yes	No
Cirrhosis/carcinoma	No	Yes	Yes	Yes	No

by consumption of contaminated foods (raw seafood) or water. Although hepatitis E virus (HEV) causes more serious infections in pregnant women, neither HAV nor HEV have a high mortality rate.

Hepatitis B, C, and D viruses are transmitted through contact with infected blood, or blood products, and have a more insidious onset than does HAV. Sharing needles, acupuncture, tattooing, and body piercing are high-risk activities associated with acquiring viral hepatitis. HBV can also be transmitted in other body fluids, such as semen, breast milk, and saliva. Hepatitis D virus (HDV, called the "delta agent") cannot replicate without a helper virus, HBV. The combination of HDV with active HBV infection results in a fulminant hepatitis infection.

HCV, previously called "non-A, non-B hepatitis," was difficult to detect since it cannot be grown in tissue culture. Blood transfusions were a major cause of "non-A, non-B hepatitis" until diagnostic tests for HCV were developed to screen blood and blood products as is done routinely for HBV. HCV infection results in continual damage to the liver cells and a constant repair process that is associated with primary hepatocellular carcinoma.

The differentiating features of the best-known viral hepatitis viruses are listed in Table 22.2.

HBV damages the liver because of an immune-mediated response from the host. HBV attaches to hepatocytes by its glycoproteins and penetrates liver cells. Partially double-stranded DNA of the virus becomes completely double-stranded, and the viral genome is integrated into the hepatocyte, where it may remain latent. Viral DNA is transcribed and encodes for HBV B core antigen (HBcAg) and e antigen (HBeAg), polymerase, and viral proteins. Cell-mediated immunity and inflammation result in symptoms and destruction of the infected cells. HBcAg stimulates T cells; however, if the T-cell response is insufficient, the infection may become chronic. Chronic infections are defined as symptoms that last more than 6 months with the persistence of surface antigen (HBsAg) in the blood. Infants with less cellular immunity are unable to eradicate the infection as well as are adults. They experience less damage to their liver cells but are more likely to shed the virus for longer periods of time and become chronic carriers.

Neutralization antibody can protect the liver from further damage, but excess antigen can overwhelm the amount of antibody. Immune complexes of antigen and antibody can lead to hypersensitivity reactions, such as vasculitis, rash, arthritis, and renal damage. As the infection resolves, the liver parenchyma regenerates, but permanent liver damage occurs with chronic or fulminant infections. The majority of patients with HBV have subclinical infections, with approximately 30% developing clinical hepatitis with jaundice. Fulminant hepatic failure occurs in <1% of patients. Approximately 5–10% of patients with HBV infection become chronic carriers (remain HBsAg-positive). Most of these patients do not have a history of clinically evident acute hepatitis.

22.6. TREATMENT AND PREVENTION

Our patient was given supportive care, and advised to avoid further injury to his liver. There is no antiviral therapy for acute hepatitis infections. The goal of therapy for chronic HBV is to suppress the viral replication below the threshold of liver injury. Patients with HBV DNA levels of 10^5–10^6 virions/mL, ALT levels twice the normal level, and histologic evidence of liver injury are candidates for antiviral therapy. Interferon-α and nucleoside analogs are currently available for treatment of patients with chronic HBV. About 30% of persons with HBV have no signs or symptoms of infection and require no intervention.

Because there is no treatment for acute hepatitis, prevention becomes more important. HBV vaccine is the best protection. It is advised that all newborns be vaccinated at birth, 1–2 months, and 6 months. Persons who were not vaccinated at birth should consider taking the series of three vaccinations, especially if they are in the high-risk groups for HBV infection. Persons with multiple sexual partners, men who have sex with men, injection drug users, household contacts of chronically infected persons, infants born to infected mothers, hemodialysis patients, and healthcare and public safety workers are considered at high risk. It is important for healthcare workers to observe "universal blood and body fluid precautions" to protect both the patient and themselves. Wearing personal protective equipment (PPE), such as gloves, gown, and eye protection, and appropriate handling and disposing of needles and other sharp instruments are required in the healthcare setting. Hepatitis B immune globulin (HBIG) can be given in the event of a healthcare worker exposure or a baby born to an antigen positive mother. Post-exposure prophylaxis consists of HBV vaccination plus HBIG. Vaccination should occur as soon as possible after exposure (ideally within 12 h).

Similarly, immunoglobulin prophylaxis is advised for close contacts of patients with HAV, to be administered within 2 weeks of coming in contact with the infected person. Vaccination for HAV is available as a two-dose regimen, and it is recommended for those traveling to countries where HAV is common. There is no prophylaxis or vaccine for HCV or HEV.

22.7. ADDITIONAL POINTS

■ Following immunization to HBV, only HBV surface antibody (HBsAb) will be present. Since the vaccine does not contain core or e antigen, no antibody to these will be detected unless the person had a natural infection with HBV. Post-vaccination testing for serologic response is not recommended for infants, children, and adolescents. Testing for immunity is advised only for persons whose subsequent clinical management depends on knowledge of their immune status (dialysis patients and staff, infants born to antigen-positive mothers, those with HIV infection). Post-vaccination testing may be done in those persons with occupational exposure to determine appropriate post-exposure prophylaxis.

■ HBV is most common in 20–49-year-old persons since routine vaccination has reduced the incidence of infection in children and adolescents.

■ Acute HBV can progress to chronic infection. The chance of progression is related to the age of the patient at the time of infection. Perinatally acquired infection usually results in chronic infection. This is commonly seen in China and other parts of Asia. In contrast, <10% of adults who acquire HBV infection will develop chronic infection. In patients with chronic HBV infection, HBsAg remains positive, and although usually asymptomatic, these individuals are at risk for the development of cirrhosis and hepatocellular carcinoma.

■ Approximately 80% of patients exposed to HCV have no signs or symptoms. However, 55–85% of persons infected with HCV progress to chronic infection. Death may result from chronic liver disease, and liver damage due to HCV is the leading indication for a liver transplant.

SUGGESTED READING

CDC, A comprehensive immunization strategy to eliminate transmission of hepatitis B virus infection in the United States, *MMWR* **54**(RR-16):1–39 (2005).

CDC, *Hepatitis Fact Sheets*, www.cdc.gov/hepatitis.

CDC, *Hepatitis Frequently Asked Questions*, www.cdc.gov/ncidod/diseases/hepatitis/.

WONG, S. N. AND A. S. LOK, Treatment of hepatitis B: Who, when, and how? *Arch. Intern. Med.* **166**:9–12 (2006).

Fever of Unknown Origin in a Traveler

23.1. PATIENT HISTORY

A 34 year-old male resident of Massachusetts presented to the hospital emergency department with a two-week history of recurrent intermittent fevers, chills, headache, and myalgia. Symptoms started one week after he returned from a two week trip in June to Peru, Colombia, Venezuela, and Brazil. He stayed in major cities, slept in modern hotels, and did not travel to rural areas or eat meals outside his hotel. He admitted to being inconsistent about taking his antimalarial prophylactic medications while traveling. He reports that he is normally in excellent health, has no underlying medical conditions, and takes no medications routinely. He is married and reports that he is monogamous and had no sexual contact with new partners during travel. He lives in a rural area in Massachusetts and frequently walks in the wooded areas around his home. Findings on physical exam were unremarkable except for mild hepatosplenomegaly and a fever of 40°C (104°F), heart rate of 110 beats/min, and blood pressure of 120/70 mm Hg.

23.2. DIFFERENTIAL DIAGNOSIS

A number of factors should be considered when evaluating this patient. He has recently traveled, and 20–25% of travelers report an illness on

Medical Microbiology for the New Curriculum: A Case-Based Approach, by Roberta B. Carey, Mindy G. Schuster, and Karin L. McGowan.
Copyright © 2008 John Wiley & Sons, Inc.

their return. In addition, he lives in a rural area of Massachusetts, a state known to be endemic for Lyme disease and babesiosis, both of which are acquired through a tick bite. He may also have an infection common in nontravelers such as community-acquired pneumonia, urinary tract infection, a viral syndrome, or bacteremia, all of which are characterized by fever.

When evaluating a febrile patient who has recently traveled, one should ask about pre-travel immunizations and antimalarial chemoprophylaxis. Besides their travel history (departure and return dates, exact travel itinerary), one should also obtain an exposure history from the patient (mosquito and insect bites, use of insect repellents, animal exposure, freshwater swimming, raw or undercooked foods consumed, untreatedwater exposure, sexual encounters).

Incubation time can be somewhat helpful. Infections with a short incubation (<10 days) include dengue, ehrlichiosis, human immunodeficiency virus (HIV), malaria, typhoid fever, and Yellow fever. Illnesses with an incubation period within 1 month include hepatitis viruses A, C, and E; amebic liver abscess; and leishmaniasis, schistosomiasis, coccidioidomycosis, and cytomegalovirus. Infections associated with longer incubation periods include hepatitis B, amebic liver abscess, and tuberculosis.

Infectious Causes

Fever of unknown origin (FUO) can be caused by any of the infectious agents listed below.

Bacteria

> *Borrelia burgdorferi* (Lyme disease)
> *Borrelia recurrentis*
> *Brucella* spp.
> *Coxiella burnetti* (Q fever)
> *Francisella tularensis*
> *Leptospira interrogans* (leptospirosis)
> *Mycobacterium tuberculosis*
> *Neisseria meningitidis*
> *Salmonella* spp.

Viruses

> Arbovirus [dengue fever, Yellow fever, Mayaro (togavirus) fever]
> Cytomegalovirus
> Epstein–Barr virus
> Human Immunodeficiency virus (HIV)
> Hepatitis A, B, C, and E
> Viral hemorrhagic fevers

Fungi

Coccidioides immitis

Cryptococcus neoformans

Histoplasma capsulatum

Parasites

Babesia spp.

Entamoeba histolytica (amebic liver abscess)

Leishmania spp.

Plasmodium spp. (malaria)

Schistosoma spp.

Trypanosoma cruzi (Chagas' disease; American trypanosomiasis)

Other Infectious Causes

Ehrlichia spp.

Rickettsia spp. (tick typhus, Rocky Mountain Spotted Fever)

CLINICAL CLUES

? Travel to a malarious area, but patient took malaria prophylaxis? You still need to think about malaria; prophylaxis is not 100% effective.

? Patient with intense myalgias and headache along with fever? Think dengue fever, also known as "breakbone fever."

? Patient with a normal pulse despite fever? Think *Salmonella,* an intracellular organism. Sometimes patients infected with intracellular organisms have a normal pulse despite high fever.

? Eosinophilia? Think migrating parasites: schistosomiasis, filaria, or strongyloides.

? Swimming in potentially infected water? Think of schistosomiasis or leptospirosis.

? Patient sexually active with new partners during travel? Look carefully for any genital lesions, rash, or lymphadenopathy indicative of a sexually transmitted disease such as herpes simplex, syphilis, or HIV.

? Patient with sore throat, lymphadenopathy, maculopapular rash, headache, and fever? Consider acute HIV infection.

23.3. LABORATORY TESTS

Because optimal treatment of malaria requires rapid case identification, and because of the life-threatening nature of both malaria and typhoid fever, initial laboratory tests for both diseases should be performed immediately. In the United States, the leading cause of death in patients with malaria is delay in diagnosis and treatment. To rule out malaria and babesiosis, thick and thin blood smears should be performed. Peripheral blood can be submitted in anticoagulant tubes if the specimen will reach the laboratory within 2 h. Tubes containing EDTA (ethylenediaminetetraacetic acid) or heparin are preferred if blood is to be examined for parasites. If initial smears are negative and malaria is still suspected, smears should be repeated every 12 h for 2–3 days. Thick and thin blood smears should be stained with Giemsa or Wright's stains. The thick smears are the most sensitive because of the larger amount of blood that is concentrated on the smear (20–40×). RBCs are lysed on the thick smears, making them more difficult to read, but thick smears are superior to thin smears for detecting low levels of parasitemia, particularly during relapse or recrudescence. Thin blood smears are methanol-fixed prior to staining so that the RBCs remain intact. Thin films are considered more specific for *Plasmodium* species identification because morphologic features of the organism and the infected RBCs are more easily visualized using thin smears. The thin smears are also preferred when estimating the percent parasitemia because the organisms are easier to see and count.

The percent parasitemia should be calculated in every positive blood smear. This percentage is an indicator of disease severity and can be used as a prognostic indicator following treatment. For this reason, quantitation of parasitemia should be repeated at 6, 12, and 24 h after starting chemotherapy. Parasitemia $\geq$ 5% is considered severe malaria, and many institutions admit patients to the ICU when the parasitemia reaches this level, particularly pediatric hospitals.

When using thick and thin blood smears for diagnosis, speciation of *Plasmodium* is achieved by examining microscopic morphologic features of both the parasite and the infected RBC. With infected RBCs, the erythrocyte size and the presence of stippling or dots are noted. Morphologic features of the *Plasmodium* parasite include number of stages seen; number of nuclei; ameboid, serrated, band, or basket trophozoites; numbers and shape of schizonts; malarial pigment; and the shape of gametocytes. *Plasmodium* should always be identified to the species level, because it will impact on the therapy choices.

While microscopy is still considered the method of choice for diagnosing malaria, it requires considerable technical expertise for correct blood smear preparation and staining as well as smear examination and interpretation. In nonendemic countries, this level of expertise is often difficult to achieve. A number of rapid test kits are now available to detect malarial antigens or enzymes directly from blood. They use a dipstick or cassette format, and results are available in less than 10 min (Fig. 23.1). Recently, FDA-approved for use in the United States, these kits offer an alternative when reliable microscopic identification is not available. In addition, they can be used as an adjunct to microscopy, offering a rapid preliminary diagnosis while thick and thin blood films are being prepared and stained. At the present time, these tests are costly and their accuracy needs to be improved, particularly for the diagnosis of *P. ovale*. Several polymerase chain reaction (PCR) assays have also been developed for the diagnosis of malaria, and while PCR is more sensitive than microscopy, it is expensive and requires a specialized laboratory and personnel, which are seldom

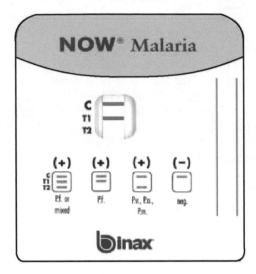

FIGURE 23.1 Rapid test for malaria.

available at all times. At the present time it appears to be an impractical way for clinical laboratories to diagnose malaria. Serology tests available for the diagnosis of malaria are not for the diagnosis of acute disease but are used for the detection of past infection.

For typhoid fever, blood (×3) and stool cultures should be performed. Other initial lab tests should include a complete blood cell count with differential, platelet count, liver function tests, urinalysis and urine culture, chest x-ray, and tuberculin skin test. A sample of acute serum (red-topped tube) should be frozen and stored when the patient is initially evaluated. A number of serology tests will require an acute and convalescent serum pair taken 4 weeks apart. If initial considerations such as malaria and typhoid fever prove to be negative, then serology tests can be ordered using the stored sera. Specific serology tests would need to be performed to make the diagnosis of rickettsial disease, HIV, dengue fever, leptospirosis, Lyme disease, ehrlichiosis, Yellow fever, hepatitis, and viral hemorrhagic fevers.

23.4. RESULTS

Laboratory tests revealed a WBC count of $4900/mm^3$ with 18% neutrophils, 60% band forms, and 22% lymphocytes; a hematocrit of 34%; and a platelet count of $59,000/mm^3$. Thick and thin blood films were positive for *Plasmodium vivax* with 3% parasitemia (Figs. 23.2, 23.3). Twenty-four hours following initiation of therapy, repeat smears were negative for parasites. Antiparasitic susceptibility of malarial strains is a research tool performed at specialized centers but is not available in routine clinical laboratories, particularly in nonendemic countries.

Blood cultures (×3) and stool and urine cultures were negative, and stool sent for ova and parasite examination was also negative. Liver function tests, urinalysis, chest x-ray, and tuberculin skin test were all within

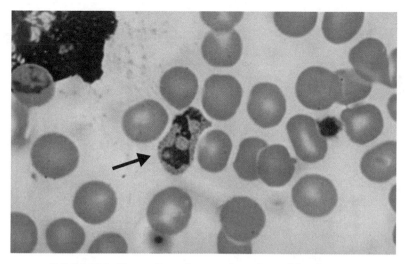

FIGURE 23.2 *Plasmodium vivax* trophozoite on blood smear.

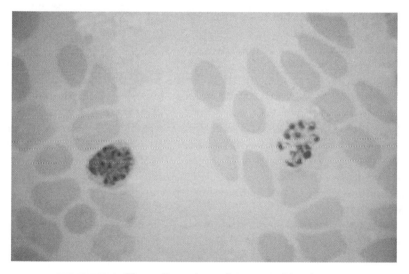

FIGURE 23.3 *Plasmodium vivax* schizonts in blood smear.

normal limits. Additional serology tests were not ordered, and the stored acute serum was discarded.

23.5. PATHOGENESIS

Although endemic malaria was eradicated from the United States in the 1940s, malaria continues to be a health problem for U.S. residents who travel to areas where malaria exists (Fig. 23.4). Endemic transmission of malaria occurs in parts of Central and South America, Africa, Asia, the Middle East, Hispañola (Dominican Republic and Haiti), and Oceania. Immigrants and travelers may present with symptoms days to weeks after returning from malarious areas. Malaria can also be acquired without

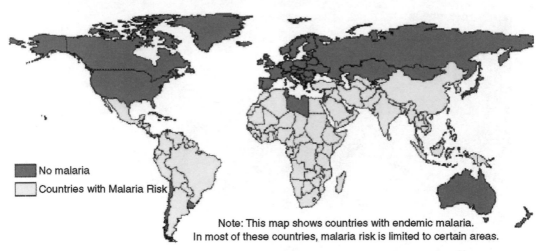

No malaria

Countries with Malaria Risk

Note: This map shows countries with endemic malaria. In most of these countries, malaria risk is limited to certain areas.

FIGURE 23.4 Malaria endemic countries, 2003.

travel exposure by either congenital infection, exposure to contaminated blood or blood products, or local mosquito-borne transmission.

Four species of *Plasmodium* cause malaria in humans: *P. falciparum*, *P. vivax*, *P. malariae*, and *P. ovale*. They differ in their life cycles and ability to parasitize erythrocytes, which affects the cyclical nature of their clinical symptoms and the severity of the disease. The interval from exposure to symptoms ranges from 9–14 days for *P. falciparum*, *P. vivax*, and *P. ovale* and over 40 days for *P. malariae*. *P. vivax* and *P. ovale* selectively infect immature erythrocytes (reticulocytes), and *P. malariae* infects only older erythrocytes. *P. falciparum* can infect red cells of all ages, and this leads to a heavy burden of infected cells. Most deaths are caused by *P. falciparum* because of its ability to parasitize a large population of red cells and cause fulminant disease.

Malarial parasites are injected into humans with the bite of an infected mosquito. The sporozoites in the salivary gland of the mosquito travel to the human liver, where they develop into merozoites. The parasites remain in the liver 1–2 weeks before the infected hepatocytes rupture and release merozoites into the bloodstream. In patients with *P. vivax* or *P. ovale* infections, some of the organisms remain latent in the liver for months or years. The merozoites in the bloodstream infect the erythrocytes and develop from ring forms to ameboid trophozoites to schizonts within 48 h, except for *P. malariae*, whose cycle takes 72 h. The schizonts rupture, releasing merozoites that infect other red cells. A subset of the merozoites differentiates into the sexual forms called gametocytes. The sexual forms are swallowed by the anopheles mosquitoes when they feed, and they fertilize and form zygotes that differentiate into ookinetes that burrow into the midgut wall of the mosquito. There they develop into oocysts that rupture, releasing the sporozoites that migrate to the salivary gland of the mosquito, and the cycle starts again as seen in Fig. 23.5.

P. falciparum has the ability to sequester in deep-vein microvasculature in the heart, lung, brain, liver, kidney, dermis, bone marrow, or placenta. There the parasites can avoid filtration and destruction in the spleen. The

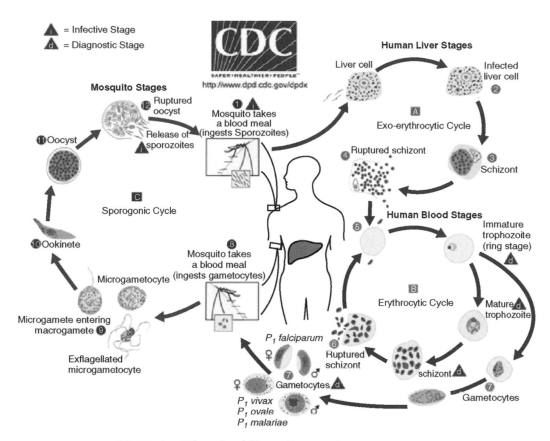

FIGURE 23.5 Life cycle of *Plasmodium* species.

late trophozoite and schizont forms of *P. falciparum* insert an antigen into the red cell membrane, causing the red cells to adhere to the vascular endothelium. The trophozoite and schizont forms are sequestered in the liver and spleen and are not seen in the peripheral blood of patients with *P. falciparum* when a microscopic exam of the blood is done to diagnose malaria. The laboratory diagnosis is based on detecting numerous delicate ring forms (Fig. 23.6) or an occasional banana-shaped gametocyte (Fig. 23.7). Sequestration of parasites stimulates production of cytokines, such as tumor necrosis factor (TNFα), which upregulates adhesion molecules, leading to more sequestration and local oxygen deprivation. *P. malariae*, *P. vivax*, and *P. ovale* do not exhibit sequestration. All parasitic forms are seen in a peripheral blood smear of a patient with these *Plasmodium* species, and their disease is more benign with the absence of microvasculature obstruction and cytokine effects.

Cerebral malaria (CM) is the most severe form of disease associated with *P. falciparum* malaria. It occurs almost exclusively in children and is the major cause of death and long-term sequelae (neurologic abnormalities, poor verbal skills, difficulty walking). CM results when sludging of parasitized RBCs occurs in the capillaries and microvessels of the brain. Seizures occur in 66% of patients with CM, and the mortality rate is 15–50%. In addition to the expected symptoms of fever, chills, and

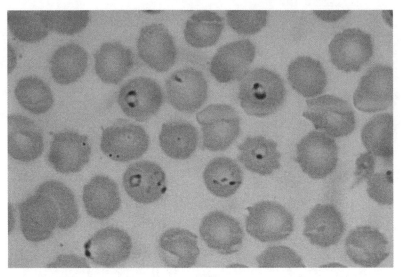

FIGURE 23.6 *Plasmodium falciparum* ring stage on blood smear.

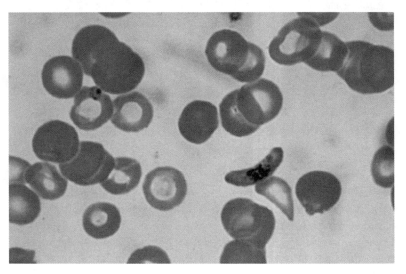

FIGURE 23.7 *Plasmodium falciparum* banana-shaped gametocyte.

rigors, patients with *P. falciparum* may have nausea, vomiting, and diarrhea. Heavy parasitemia in the kidneys may cause intravascular hemolysis and hemoglobinuria, which results in acute renal failure, nephritic syndrome, and death, commonly referred to as "blackwater fever."

23.6. TREATMENT AND PREVENTION

Malaria is a nationally notifiable disease, and all cases should be reported to the state public health department, who forward the information to the Centers for Disease Control and Prevention (CDC). Clinicians at CDC

Malaria Hotline provide advice on the diagnosis and treatment of malaria 24 h/day (770-488-7788 weekdays; 770-488-7100 nights, weekends, and holidays).

Treatment of malaria should not be initiated until the diagnosis has been confirmed by a positive blood smear or other laboratory test. In extreme conditions, if there is a strong clinical suspicion and the patient is severely ill with little opportunity to get a timely laboratory confirmation, therapy may be started. Therapy is guided by three factors: the clinical status of the patient, the *Plasmodium* species, and the drug susceptibility of the parasite as determined by the geographic location where the infection was acquired.

Patients diagnosed with uncomplicated malaria can be effectively treated with oral therapy. Chloroquine remains the drug of choice for our patient's *P. vivax* infection, and for *P. ovale*, unless the infection was acquired in Papua New Guinea or Indonesia, where chloroquine-resistant *P. vivax* has been documented. Chloroquine is also the drug of choice for all *P. malariae* infections, and for *P. falciparum* infections acquired in areas without chloroquine-resistant strains, which includes Central America, Hispañola, and parts of the Middle East. Because areas with chloroquine resistance are changing, one should refer to the CDC Yellow Book or call the CDC Malaria Hotline for the most up-to-date information. Treatment options for chloroquine-resistant *P. falciparum* infections are quinine sulfate plus deoxycycline, tetracycline, or clindamycin; or atovaquone–proguanil. Mefloquine, a third agent prescribed, has a higher risk of side effects. Patients with *P. vivax*, *P. ovale*, or *P. malariae* can usually be treated as outpatients. Because of the higher associated morbidity and mortality, patients with *P. falciparum* should be treated in the hospital initially to monitor for complications. The mortality rate associated with *P. falciparum* can be as high as 3–4%, and is usually a result of a delay in diagnosis or missed diagnosis. Blood smears should be repeated every 12 h on therapy until the parasitemia is below 1%.

In addition to treating the blood phase of malaria, our patient must also receive therapy to eradicate organisms that remain viable but dormant in the liver. Our patient will require 14 days of primaquine phosphate. However, this therapy may cause hemolytic anemia in persons with glucose-6-phosphate dehydrogenase (G6PD) deficiency, and the patient must be screened for this enzyme deficiency prior to receiving primaquine therapy.

If parasitemia exceeds 5% and symptoms of severe disease are present, the patient should receive parenteral antimalarial therapy. Quinidine gluconate is the only recommended agent available in the United States. This drug is cardiotoxic, and blood pressure must be monitored carefully. An exchange transfusion may be considered in infants and young children with a parasitemia greater than 10% to remove infected red cells and toxins, metabolites, and cytokines.

Travelers must be aware that acquired immunity is short-lived without continual re-exposure to infection and that they are susceptible to reinfection. No vaccine is currently available, and no method can protect completely against the risk for contracting malaria. In addition, restrictions are placed on donating blood for one year following return from a

TABLE 23.1.	Comparison of Characteristics of the Four Species of *Plasmodium*			
	P. falciparum	*P. vivax*	*P. ovale*	*P. malariae*
Red cells infected	All stages	Immature	Immature	Mature
Forms in peripheral blood	Rings, gametocytes	Rings, trophozoites, schizonts, gametocytes	Rings, trophozoites, schizonts, gametocytes	Rings, trophozoites, schizonts, gametocytes
Cycle time in peripheral blood (h)	48	48	48	72
Disease	Fulminant	Benign	Benign	Benign
Latent in liver	No	Yes	Yes	No
Forms sequestered in deep vein	Yes	No	No	No
Primary therapy	Chloroquine	Chloroquine + primaquine	Chloroquine + primaquine	Chloroquine
Chloroquine resistance	Yes	Yes	Yes	No

malarious area. Key differential characteristics of the four species of *Plasmodium* are listed in Table 23.1.

Chemoprophylaxis before, during, and after exposure to malaria is the primary method of preventing or suppressing symptoms caused by the malarial parasite in the blood. Malaria prophylaxis with chloroquine is used for travel to areas free of chloroquine-resistant *P. falciparum*. For travel to areas with chloroquine-resistant *P. falciparum* (Africa, parts of Asia), prophylactic options include mefloquine, atovaquone–proguanil, doxycycline, and primaquine. Prophylaxis is started 1–2 weeks prior to departure to ensure adequate protective levels in the blood before exposure. Chemoprophylaxis should be continued for 4 weeks after leaving the malarious area. One of the most common reasons why patients acquire malaria is their failure to continue prophylaxis after they return home. The CDC Travelers' Health Website http://cdc.gov/travel updates locations where chloroquine- and mefloquine-resistant malaria have been documented. For persons who have had prolonged exposure to *P. vivax* and/or *P. ovale*, a terminal prophylaxis with primaquine decreases the risk of relapse in those species that may be latent in the liver. It is very important that all persons taking primaquine have a normal glucose-6-phosphate dehydrogenase (G6PD) level prior to initiating therapy.

Wearing protective clothing, sleeping under insecticide-treated mosquito nets, and using insect repellent with DEET (*N*,*N*-diethyl-*m*-toluamide) are personal protective measures in addition to taking chemoprophylaxis that should be discussed with travelers to countries where malaria is endemic.

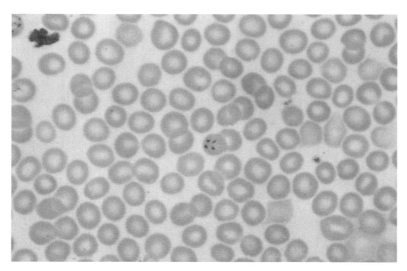

FIGURE 23.8 Tetrad-shaped trophozoite of *Babesia microti*.

23.7. ADDITIONAL POINTS

■ Malaria during pregnancy can be an extremely serious disease. Malaria prophylaxis and treatment are both complicated by pregnancy because of adverse effects of medications in the mother and fetus. Pregnant women develop malarial parasitemia and a higher degree of parasitemia more frequently than do nonpregnant women. Malaria adversely affects both the mother and the fetus. There is an increase in maternal mortality and morbidity [acute respiratory distress syndrome (ARDS), massive hemolysis, disseminated intravascular coagulopathy (DIC), hypoglycemia, acute renal failure] as well as an increase in the incidence of abortion, stillbirth, prematurity, fetal distress, intrauterine growth retardation, and reduced birth weight.

■ On occasion, people with no risk factors (e.g., history of travel outside the United States, injection drug use, blood transfusion, or previous malaria infection) are diagnosed with acute malaria. This is called cryptic or locally acquired malaria. Sources of such infections include infected anophelese mosquitoes transported by aircraft to nonendemic areas (airport malaria), and unrecognized malaria infections among recent immigrants, migrant workers, or travelers from malaria-endemic countries. Anophelese mosquitoes capable of transmitting malaria exist throughout the United States, except Alaska.

■ Babesiosis has a clinical presentation resembling malaria, and persons who do not have a functional spleen are more likely to be infected and have more severe disease. *Babesia microti* is the most common species seen in the Northeast (Martha's Vineyard and other parts of New England) and the U.S. Midwest, where the organisms infect deer, rodents, and cattle. The parasites are transmitted by the bite of an *Ixodes* tick. Intracellular ring forms similar to *P. falciparum* can be seen in the peripheral blood smear of an infected person. However, extracellular *Babesia* ring forms may also be observed. The unique tetrad appearance of *Babesia* in the infected erythrocyte and the lack of malarial pigment distinquish babesiosis from malaria (Fig. 23.8). A good history of patient travel to an endemic location and a positive smear solidify the diagnosis. Patients are treated with clindamycin and quinine, and those with mild disease may recover without specific therapy.

SUGGESTED READING

CDC *Treatment Guidelines*, www.cdc.gov/malaria/pdf/treatmenttable.pdf.

CDC, *Yellow Book. Health Information for International Travel, 2005–2006.*

MOODY, A., Rapid diagnostic tests for malaria parasites, *Clin. Microbiol. Rev.* **15**:66–78 (2002).

Student with Fever, Lymphadenopathy and Hepatosplenomegaly

24.1. PATIENT HISTORY

The patient is a 20 year-old male college student. He was seen at student health for fever, headache, rash, and sore throat two weeks ago. At that time he was noted to have a temperature of 38.6° C (101.5°F) and to have a faint, erythematous, maculopapular rash on his trunk and a slightly erythematous pharynx without any tonsillar exudates. His exam was otherwise unremarkable. A rapid strep test and a monospot test were both negative, and he was discharged with a diagnosis of "viral syndrome," and told to return if the symptoms did not resolve. Now, two weeks later, the fever, headache, and sore throat have resolved, but he has noticed some swollen lymph nodes. His physical exam was notable for nontender cervical and axillary lymphadenopathy, and mild hepatosplenomegaly.

24.2. DIFFERENTIAL DIAGNOSIS

For any patient with acute onset of headache and fever, the diagnosis of bacterial meningitis should be entertained. Our patient's symptoms of fever, rash, and sore throat are somewhat nonspecific, but suggest a viral infection. Many viruses can cause fever and rash, including enteroviruses, hepatitis viruses, cytomegalovirus, parvovirus, measles, rubella, and

Medical Microbiology for the New Curriculum: A Case-Based Approach, by Roberta B. Carey, Mindy G. Schuster, and Karin L. McGowan.
Copyright © 2008 John Wiley & Sons, Inc.

roseola. Secondary syphilis should be considered as well. The presence of sore throat should raise the suspicion of Epstein–Barr virus infection. Headache is common in patients with febrile viral illnesses, but can also be a sign of aseptic meningitis. The agents that should be considered as a cause of our patient's symptoms are listed below.

Infectious Causes

Bacteria

Borrelia burgdorferi

Ehrlichia spp.

Neisseria gonorrhoeae

Neisseria meningitidis

Rickettsia rickettsii

Staphylococcal or streptococcal toxic shock syndromes

Streptococcus pyogenes (group A strep)

Treponema pallidum

Viruses

Cytomegalovirus (CMV)

Enterovirus

Epstein–Barr virus (EBV)

Hepatitis A, B, C

Herpes simplex virus (HSV)

Human herpesvirus 6 (HHV-6)

Human immunodeficiency virus (HIV)

Parvovirus B19

Rubella

Fungi

No fungi are likely causes of these symptoms.

Parasites

Toxoplasma gondii

Noninfectious Causes

Bechet's disease

Drug reaction

Lymphoma

Vasculitis

CLINICAL CLUES

? A mononucleosis-like syndrome and oral thrush (candidiasis)? Think acute HIV infection.

? Fever, rash, and lymphadenopathy? These nonspecific symptoms are associated with many viral infections.

? A mononucleosis-like syndrome in a traveler returning from areas with high endemic rates of HIV? Think acute HIV infection.

24.3. LABORATORY DIAGNOSIS

The initial laboratory tests ordered to evaluate this patient included a complete blood count and differential, prothrombin time, platelet count, electrolytes, blood urea nitrogen (BUN), creatinine, erythrocyte sedimentation rate, C-reactive protein, and a complete battery of liver function tests (LFTs) including albumin, serum bilirubin, cholesterol, total protein, alkaline phosphatase, alanine aminotransferase (ALT), aspartate aminotransferase (AST), and γ-glutamyltranspeptidase (GGT). Serum was obtained for serology testing for hepatitis A, B, and C; *Toxoplasma gondii*; Epstein–Barr virus (specific antibody); CMV, parvovirus B19; HHV-6; rapid plasma reagin (RPR) for syphilis, and an enzyme immunoassay (EIA) for HIV. In addition, polymerase chain reaction (PCR) testing was ordered for HSV.

While awaiting results on many of the laboratory tests above, the EIA for HIV-1/2 performed on this patient's serum was reported as weakly reactive. During acute HIV infections, these tests are typically nonreactive or weakly reactive because the patient is just beginning to mount a detectable antibody response. HIV-1/2 EIA antibody tests are more than 99% sensitive and specific, but some false-positive test results do occur. Because of this, all positive EIA results must be confirmed by a second test, such as a Western blot. Guidelines for HIV testing vary from country to country, but in the United States, initial screening is performed with an EIA for antibodies to HIV-1/2. Specimens with a nonreactive result are considered HIV-1/2-negative. Specimens with a reactive EIA result are retested in duplicate, and if either duplicate is reactive, the specimen is reported as repeatedly reactive. Confirmatory testing with a supplemental test is then performed (e.g., Western blot), and if positive, the specimen is considered HIV-positive. Screening tests possess a high degree of sensitivity, while confirmatory assays have a high specificity. The combination of the two types of tests (screening plus confirmatory) produces results that are highly accurate, and this approach is used with a number of illnesses, including Lyme disease. A variety of laboratory tests are available to diagnose and/or monitor HIV infection, and these are listed below. For all HIV-related tests, patient consent must be obtained in order for testing to be performed.

HIV EIA (ELISA)

Antibodies to HIV-1/2 are detected by assays known as enzyme-linked immunosorbent assays (ELISA or EIA) performed using patient serum.

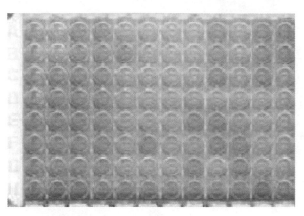

FIGURE 24.1 ELISA plate.

Use of EIA as a screening test for HIV was initiated in 1985, when a highly sensitive method was needed to screen the blood supply in the United States. HIV antibody tests are more than 99% sensitive, so that the only infected patients who are not detected are those tested within the first few weeks after acquiring the infection. The specificity of HIV antibody tests is also better than 99%, but some false-positive tests do occur in multiparous women; recent recipients of influenza or hepatitis B vaccines; those with hematological malignancies, multiple myeloma, primary biliary cirrhosis, or alcoholic hepatitis; and those who have received multiple transfusions. To perform an EIA test, the wells of plastic microtiter plates are coated with recombinant viral proteins (antigens), which stick to the plastic. When serum from an infected patient is added to the well, HIV antibodies bind to the proteins, becoming attached to the plate. After the plate is rinsed, the bound antibodies are detected by a second antibody that is linked to an enzyme. The second antibody binds to human anti-HIV antibodies. The antigen–antibody–enzyme complex is then detected by adding a substrate to the plate that turns yellow when it reacts with the enzyme (Fig. 24.1). With EIA technology, many specimens can be tested quickly and economically, and the microtiter plates are read by instruments, thus requiring less personnel time.

Western Blot

While not as sensitive as an EIA assay, the Western blot is more specific and allows one to identify the specific HIV proteins to which the antibodies are reacting. It is the principal HIV confirmatory test used worldwide. Western blot assays show antibodies directed against individual viral proteins. In an HIV Western blot, proteins of HIV-1 undergo electrophoresis into a gel where they are separated according to their molecular weight (size) and charge. The separated proteins are then transferred onto a thin nitrocellulose strip. To perform the test, patient serum is added to the strip and anti-HIV antibodies will bind to the separate HIV antigens. A detection enzyme is then added, which binds to the antibodies, and then a chemical is added that changes color when it binds to the protein–antibody–enzyme complex. The end result is a series of shaded bands (Fig. 24.2). Glycoprotein bands are labeled "gp" with their corresponding molecular

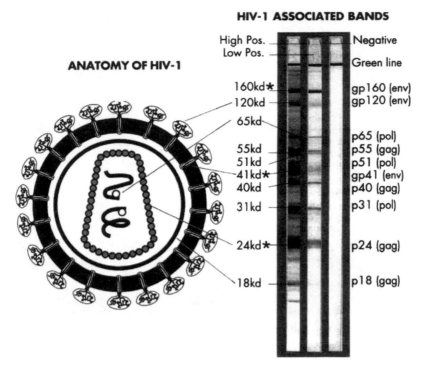

HIV-1 ASSOCIATED BANDS

ANATOMY OF HIV-1

High Pos. — Negative
Low Pos. —
Green line

160kd* — gp160 (env)
120kd — gp120 (env)
65kd —
p65 (pol)
55kd — p55 (gag)
51kd — p51 (pol)
41kd* — gp41 (env)
40kd — p40 (gag)
31kd — p31 (pol)

24kd* — p24 (gag)

18kd — p18 (gag)

FIGURE 24.2 Western blot of HIV-1 showing bands associated with viral structures.

weight in thousands (e.g., gp120/160, gp41), and protein bands are labeled "p" with their molecular weight in thousands (e.g., p24, p31, p66). In 1987, the Centers for Disease Control, along with several other organizations, issued interpretation recommendations for HIV Western blot test results proposing that a positive test result be defined by the presence of any two of the following bands: p24, gp41, and gp120/160 (considered one antigen). If bands are present but the pattern does not meet the CDC criteria for positivity, the test is considered "indeterminate." If no bands are present, the test result is negative.

Rapid HIV Tests

Recently, there has been an increase in the development of rapid diagnostic tests for HIV. Rapid tests can be used in place of traditional EIA tests and are being used in sites such as physician offices, sexually transmitted disease (STD) clinics, and anonymous test sites. Rather than waiting for blood to be sent to a reference laboratory and requiring patients to return days later for test results, screening test results are available within 30 min. Rapid tests can be also be helpful in identifying HIV infection in women in labor who have not had prenatal HIV testing and when testing source patients in needlestick injuries. Rapid tests are as accurate as an EIA when performed carefully by experienced personnel, but just as with an EIA screening test, a rapid test positive result must be confirmed with a Western blot assay. At the present time, rapid tests using whole blood, oral fluid, and plasma are FDA-approved for use (Figs. 24.3, 24.4).

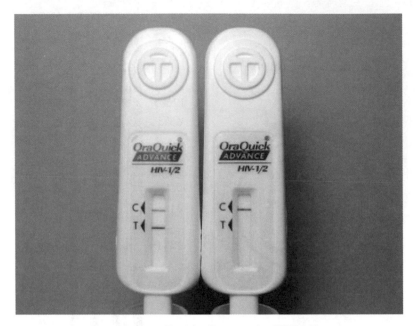

FIGURE 24.3 Rapid saliva test for HIV-1/2.

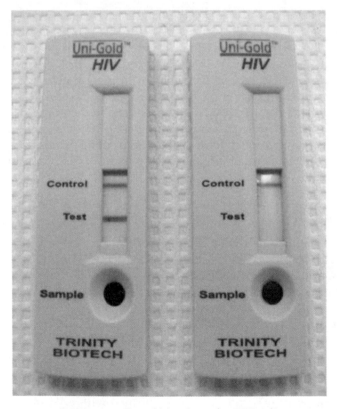

FIGURE 24.4 Rapid blood test for HIV-1/2.

CD4 Counts

The CD4 molecule is expressed on the surface of helper T lymphocytes, and it serves as the primary receptor for HIV-1 and HIV-2. The progressive loss of T helper cells is a typical finding in patients with acquired immunodeficiency syndrome (AIDS) and is an independent risk factor for progression to AIDS and death. Because it provides an estimate of the immune status of a patient, the CD4 count is an excellent indicator of a patient's risk for opportunistic infection. Opportunistic infections are rare in patients with CD4 counts above 500 cells/mm^3, but the risk increases appreciably as the CD4 count falls below 200 cells/mm^3.

In addition to being a marker for risk of opportunistic infection, the CD4 count increases in response to antiretroviral therapy. Falling CD4 is a marker of disease progression. Patients who achieve a significant CD4 cell increase in response to antiretroviral therapy have a considerably lower risk of disease progression. Current guidelines suggest that CD4 counts be measured at the time of diagnosis and every 3–6 months thereafter. If the patient is having symptoms or is ill, CD4 counts should be performed more frequently.

HIV Culture

HIV-1 can be cultured from peripheral blood mononuclear cells of infected patients. A positive culture provides direct evidence of HIV-1 infection and is recommended for (1) detecting HIV-1 in infants ≤ 18 months of age born to HIV-infected mothers, (2) diagnosis of acute HIV infection in high-risk populations, and (3) facilitating resolution of indeterminate Western blot antibody test results. Viral cultures are performed by mixing patient cells with cells from uninfected donors that have been stimulated with phytohemagglutinin. Growth of HIV-1 in culture is determined by testing culture supernatants for p24 antigen using an enzyme immunoassay. Cultures usually become positive within two weeks, but some cultures may require up to 60 days to become positive.

HIV-1 PCR (Qualitative)

This qualitative test involves amplification and detection of HIV-1 DNA from purified peripheral blood mononuclear cells and other specimens (tissue, sterile fluid) using real-time polymerase chain reaction (PCR). Assays for detecting HIV-1 DNA use PCR to amplify conserved sequences in the HIV-1 *gag* (p24) or *pol* (p31) genes. Using this method, laboratories achieve 96–99% sensitivity and specificity in PCR testing for HIV-1.

Viral Load Testing (Quantitative Plasma HIV-1 RNA Levels)

Viral load is the quantity of HIV-RNA that is in the blood or plasma. The viral load test is used to monitor the status of HIV disease, to guide beginning or changing antiretroviral therapy, and to predict the risk for disease progression. Viral load and trends in viral load are thought to be more informative for decision making regarding antiretroviral therapy than are CD4 counts. Evidence shows that keeping the viral load levels as low as possible for as long as possible decreases the complications of HIV disease and prolongs life. Because viral load tests can detect HIV more quickly than other tests can, they are also indicated for testing newborn babies whose mothers have been diagnosed with HIV or AIDS. If test results show that HIV is present in the baby's blood sample, treatment can be initiated sooner. In pregnant HIV-infected women, the viral load predicts transmission risk.

Presently there are three different viral load laboratory tests:

1. The polymerase chain reaction test (PCR) is the most common assay currently being used. Test results are reported as the number of HIV copies/per milliliter of plasma.

2. The branched chain DNA test (bDNA) is also frequently used. These test results are reported as units/mL of plasma.

3. The nucleic acid sequence-based amplification (NASBA) is less frequently used. Test results are reported as units/mL of plasma as in the bDNA test.

Because the three tests do not give exactly the same results, it is important that the same type of viral load testing be performed each time. A high viral load test result can range from 5000 to $\geq$ 1,000,000 copies/mL. A low viral load can range between 200 and 500 copies/mL. A viral load result that is "undetectable" means that the level of HIV virus in the blood is below the detection threshold of the test. Detecting a change in viral load is also important. A rising count indicates an infection that is getting worse, while a falling count indicates improvement.

An expert panel for the International AIDS Society—USA has issued guidelines indicating when viral loads should be measured. In a newly diagnosed patient, one should take two different viral load measurements 2–3 weeks apart to determine a baseline measurement. The test should be repeated every 3–6 months after that in conjunction with CD4 counts and should be repeated 4–6 weeks after starting or changing antiretroviral therapy. Current treatment guidelines suggest that anyone with a viral load over 55,000 copies/mL (bDNA test or PCR test) be offered treatment. Viral load testing should not be used for diagnosing HIV since the HIV EIA antibody test is still the preferred method for this.

Genotype Testing

Genotypic tests determine the nucleotide sequence of specific genes, or parts of genes. The most commonly used genotypic assays rely on automated DNA sequencing. Viruses that have the same gene sequence as other viruses found in nature are called "wild-type viruses." Point mutations may occur in the virus of patients who take antiretroviral agents. Genotypic testing detects the presence of mutations in a patient's virus population by identifying gene changes that differ from the wild-type genetic sequence of HIV. Genotyping indicates which drugs are not likely to be effective in reducing the viral load of the patient. Knowledge of the specific pattern of drug resistance can be helpful when choosing the treatment regimen for a patient. Drug selection based on genotyping of HIV appears to improve long-term treatment outcomes for HIV/AIDS patients.

p24 Antigen Assays

The p24 antigen assay measures the viral capsid (core) p24 protein in blood that is detectable earlier than HIV antibody during acute infection. HIV p24 antigen tests employ EIA technology with modifications to detect antigen, rather than antibody. While originally thought to be useful for early diagnosis of HIV and blood screening, the test has proven to be too insensitive. These assays are also subject to false-positive reactions due to interfering substances and immune complexes.

The primary use for the p24 antigen test is to detect antigen in supernatants from cultures that have been inoculated with cells from a patient suspected of being infected (viral culture and isolation). It is the method of choice for detecting the presence of free p24 antigen in culture.

24.4. RESULTS

This patient's EIA was repeatedly reactive, and Western blot result was positive. Physicians then ordered additional tests, and the results were as follows:

CD4 count: 350 cells/μL.

Plasma HIV RNA viral load: 623 copies/mL.

Genotype testing: Genotypic analysis of the viral polymerase (*pol*) gene predicted that the patient's virus was susceptible to most agents in three classes of antiretroviral agents: nucleoside or nucleotide analog reverse transcriptase inhibitors, nonnucleoside reverse transcriptase inhibitors, and protease inhibitors.

24.5. PATHOGENESIS

HIV enters the body via the bloodstream by contact with infected blood, through sexual intercourse, or from mother to her newborn. The virus infects dendritic cells during intercourse, travels to the lymph nodes, where it multiplies, and then enters the bloodstream. Initially the large production of virus causes a mononucleosis-like syndrome as seen in our patient, who had a flu-like illness that disappeared without intervention. After the initial burst of viral replication, the viral level in the blood declines as the virus becomes latent, but replication continues in the lymph nodes.

HIV has tropism for CD4 expressing T cells and macrophages. The infection of CD4 T-cells leads to cell death or a latent infection. When the CD4 cell population decreases, there is a loss of T-cell function with the loss of helper cells and reduced delayed hypersensitivity. Late in the disease the viral level in the blood once again increases, CD4 counts significantly decrease, and the structure of the lymph node is destroyed. When the CD4 count is <450/μL, the person is more susceptible to infections with yeasts, herpes viruses, and intracellular bacteria (*Salmonella, Listeria*). When the CD4 cell count falls below 200, severe opportunistic infections, Kaposi's sarcoma, and lymphoma may occur. In later stages, neurologic abnormalities, known as HIV dementia, further impair the infected host. HIV-1 is an enveloped, positive strand RNA virus that encodes a RNA-dependent DNA polymerase, which transcribes RNA into a copy of DNA. This is unlike most viruses that use DNA as a template to produce RNA that transcribes the message into protein.

Three major genes encode for the polyproteins, which are further cleaved to form key enzymes and structural proteins: *gag* (group-specific antigen, core and capsid protein), *pol* (polymerase, protease, integrase), and *env* (envelope glycoprotein). There are also six accessory genes to regulate replication. These principal polyproteins are the target of antiviral therapy against this virus.

HIV enters the cell by fusing with the cellular membrane of the host at specific receptor sites that have CD4 or chemokine receptors. The virus is engulfed into the cell, and viral RNA is released. Reverse transcriptase, the unique enzyme of HIV, allows viral RNA to be transcribed into complementary DNA, called the provirus. Double-stranded DNA is formed from the provirus, and an integrase enzyme splices the viral DNA into the host chromosome. Viral DNA is transcribed by the host's RNA polymerase into RNA. Messenger RNA is translated into viral structural proteins, enzymes, and envelope glycoproteins. All the building blocks are present to construct new virions, and the mature virus buds from the host cell surface and is released.

Originally HIV-1 was seen in male homosexuals, hemophiliacs, Haitians, and heroin users. The virus is similar to simian immunodeficiency virus. It is a very effective pathogen, due to the long asymptomatic phase that allows it to spread from person to person before any signs or symptoms are evident. It is capable of being transmitted to all populations via sexual contact and contaminated blood or tissues. Since 1985 in the United States, all organ and blood products have been screened for HIV infection, and this screening has almost eliminated the spread of HIV through this mechanism. Universal blood and body fluid precautions, such as those used to protect healthcare workers from hepatitis B and C, also protect against infection with HIV.

24.6. TREATMENT AND PREVENTION

The timing of initiation of treatment for HIV infection is somewhat controversial. Trials are ongoing to evaluate the optimal timing for initiation of treatment. Treatment of HIV infection is a rapidly moving and complex field, and patients should be referred to an expert in the area for treatment decisions.

When treatment is initiated, *h*ighly *a*ctive *a*ntiretroviral *t*reatment (HAART) is chosen, and the goal is to suppress the viral load (plasma HIV RNA load) to a level that is undetectable. Of utmost importance in achieving this goal is patient adherence to medications. It is felt that 95% adherence is needed to achieve an undetectable viral load in >80% of patients. Clinicians are notoriously poor judges of patient compliance or adherence. Patient education about HIV is very important. Another concern about poor adherence is the potential for the emergence of antiviral resistance.

Since it is recognized that drug-resistant virus can be transmitted during acute infection, initial treatment is guided by genotype testing of the virus, which enables evaluation of antiviral resistance. HIV drugs are used in combination. Classes include protease inhibitors (PI), nonnucleoside reverse transcriptase inhibitors (NNRTI), nucleoside or nucleotide reverse transcriptase inhibitors (NRTI), and fusion inhibitors. Side effects of HAART can be significant and may include metabolic changes such as changes in body fat (lipodystrophy) and lipid abnormalities, dysregulation of glucose metabolism, lactic acidemia, and decreases in bone mineral densities. These side effects can present significant challenges in the treatment of HIV infection.

It is important to record a history of all prior medical conditions and medications that have the potential to interact with HAART. A history of prior vaccinations is important as well. Patients should also be questioned about any history of previous opportunistic infections. They should be specifically asked about prior history of tuberculosis or a positive skin test (+PPD), due to the high chance of reactivation during HIV infection. Additionally, a full travel history should be discussed, including any residence in areas endemic for fungal infections such as coccidioidomycosis (U.S. Southwest) or histoplasmosis (Ohio or Mississippi River valley), which may also reactivate with immune suppression. A thorough history of prior sexually transmitted diseases should be taken with a discussion about risk factors for transmission. It is not uncommon for travelers to participate in riskier (unprotected) sexual activity while traveling than they might at home. All patients should be counseled about risk reduction, including the need to avoid sharing needles and to consistently use condoms during oral, vaginal, or anal sex. Because of the high viral load that often accompanies acute HIV infection, transmission may be more likely to occur at this time. Patients should be encouraged to notify all potential partners at risk for HIV. The laws on mandatory partner notification vary by state.

Patients should be questioned about the presence of fever, sweats, weight loss, difficulty swallowing, headache, visual changes, and changes in neurologic functioning. Initial physical exam requires careful attention to the skin (looking for Kaposi's sarcoma and evidence of infections), oropharynx (thrush, ulcers), lymph nodes, liver, spleen, anogenital inspection, Papanicolaou (PAP) smear for women (to screen for HPV and cervical cancer), and fundoscopic exam.

Those infected with HIV produce neutralizing antibodies, which coat the virus, but the virus remains infectious. Persistent infection of macrophages and CD4 cells allows the virus inside the cells to escape the immune system and to be protected from the environment. Although intensive research has been ongoing, there is no vaccine at this time.

24.7. ADDITIONAL POINTS

- HIV-2 is a variant of HIV-1, which is prevalent in western Africa. The U.S. blood supply is screened for the presence of both of these viruses.
- Azidothymidine (AZT), a nucleoside analog that inhibits reverse transcriptase, is given to pregnant females to reduce the risk of transmitting the virus to the fetus.

■ Absolute CD4 counts below 200 are associated with an increased risk for opportunistic infections such as *Pneumocystitis carinii* (*jiroveci*) pneumonia, esophageal candidiasis, and toxoplasmosis. Even lower CD4 counts may be associated with cryptococcal meningitis, cytomegalovirus retinitis, disseminated *Mycobacterium avium-intracellulare*, HIV wasting disease, and other opportunistic infections.

■ All whole-blood and plasma donations collected in the United States are presently being screened for HIV by nucleic acid amplification testing (NAAT). Because this test detects viral genes rather than antibodies or antigens, it is capable of detecting positives earlier in the disease and detecting more positives than antibody testing. When antibody detection was used for screening, the "window period" when the virus would be undetectable was 22 days. This period has been reduced to 12 days with the use of NAAT.

SUGGESTED READING

CDC, Revised recommendations for HIV testing of adults, adolescents, and pregnant women in healthcare settings, *MMWR* **55**(RR-14):1–17 (2006).

CDC, Epidemiology of HIV/AIDS—U.S. 1981–2005, *MMWR* **55**:589–592 (2006).

SAAG, M. S., M. HOLODNIY, D. R. KURITZKES, ET AL., HIV viral load markers in clinical practice: Recommendations of an International AIDS Society—USA Expert Panel, *Nature Med.* **2**:625–629 (1996).

Index

Medical Microbiology for the New Curriculum: A Case-Based Approach, by Roberta B. Carey, Mindy G. Schuster, and Karin L. McGowan.
Copyright © 2008 John Wiley & Sons, Inc.